Diseases of the Eye

History of Ophthalmic Medicine – Treatments and Diagnoses Described by a Surgeon and Professor of Ophthalmology in the 19th Century

By Nathaniel L. MacBride

Dean of the College of the New York Ophthalmic Hospital; Professor of Ophthalmology in the College of the New York Ophthalmic Hospital; One of the Governing Surgeons of the New York Ophthalmic Hospital; Formerly Consulting Physician to the Five Points House of Industry

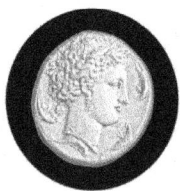

PANTIANOS
CLASSICS

Published by Pantianos Classics

ISBN-13: 978-1-78987-079-4

First published in 1897

Contents

Disclaimer

The contents of this book represent ophthalmologic medical procedures and treatments of the late nineteenth century. The publisher does not condone, advise or assume any responsibility for this book's use in any medical context.

The contents herein are presented purely for informational and historical purposes.

Preface

In preparing the following pages, the author has endeavored to set forth the results of his experience and study in a form that will prove most useful to the busy general practitioner. With this aim in view words have been used very sparingly, and only such remedies, operations, and means of diagnosis recommended as the writer believes will be found to be most useful in our present state of knowledge to the practical physician.

New York,
April, 1897

List of Remedies.

Names.	Abbreviations.
Aconitum napellus,	Acon.
Agaricus muscarius,	Agar.
Antimonium tartaricum,	Ant. Tart.
Apis mellifica,	Apis mel.
Argentum nitricum,	Argent. nit.
Arnica radix,	Arnica
Arsenicum album,	Arsenicum.
Atropine sulphate,	Atropia.
Aurum muriaticum,	Aurum mur.
Belladonna,	Bell.
Boracic acid,	Boracic ac.
Bryonia alba,	Bry.
Calcarea phosphorica,	Calc. phos.
Calcarea iodata,	Calc. iod.
Causticum,	Caust.
Cinnabaris,	Cinnabaris.
Cocaine,	Cocaine muriate.
Cuprum metallicum,	Cuprum met.
Eserine sulphate,	Eserine.
Gelsemium sempervirens,	Gels.
Hamamelis Virginica,	Hamamelis.
Helleborus niger,	Hell. nig.
Hepar sulphuris calcareum,	Hepar sulph.
Hydrobromate of Hyoscine,	Hyoscine.
Iodium,	Iodine.
Ipecacuanha	Ipecac.
Kali iodatum,	Kali iod.
Mercurius iodatus ruber,	Merc, biniod.
Mercurius cyanatus,	Merc. cyan.
Mercurius dulcis,	Merc. dulc.
Mercurius solubilis,	Merc. sol.
Mercurius corrosivus,	Merc. corr.
Nux vomica,	Nux vom.
Phosphorus,	Phos.
Pilocarpine,	Pilocarpine.
Pulsatilla nigricans,	Puls.

Rhus toxicodendron,	Rhux tox.
Scopolamine,	Scopolamine.
Sulphur,	Sulphur.
Thuja,	Thuja.
Veratrum viride,	Veratrum vir.
Zincum valerianicum,	Zinc. val.

The attenuation of the remedies recommended are expressed by the following signs: θ (the Greek letter theta) means tincture; ix (or first decimal) means that nine parts of sugar of milk, alcohol or distilled water have been added to one part of the pure medicinal substance 2x expresses the attenuation of the ix by nine, and so on up the scale. The preparation may be in the form of a powder or tablet triturate, in which case one grain is the amount prescribed; or it may be in the form of a liquid, in which case one drop is the dose indicated.

Section One

Anatomy and Physiology of the Conjunctiva, Cornea, Iris, Ciliary Body and Sclera.

Diseases of The Conjunctiva, Cornea, Iris, Ciliary Body and Sclera.

Chapter One - Anatomy and Physiology of The Conjunctiva, Cornea, Iris, Ciliary Body and Sclera

The conjunctiva is a mucous membrane which lines the eyelids and covers the anterior third of the eyeball. Its epithelium is continuous with that of the cornea. It is loosely connected with the sclera by subconjunctival tissue, which is continuous with the capsule of Tenon and with the tendons of the external ocular muscles. The palpebral portion of the conjunctiva is firmly adherent to the lids. It is reflected from the lids to the ball in the form of loose folds. The loose connection between this part of the membrane and the tissues of the orbit allows the eye great freedom of movement, and also permits of great swelling. The sac formed by the conjunctiva in passing from the lids to the ball is called the "fornix." Mucous glands are found along its course and also along the convex border of the tarsus. Diffuse adenoid tissue, lymphoid cells and circumscribed lymph follicles are found in this membrane, especially along the retrotarsal folds. To view all parts of the conjunctiva it is necessary to evert the eyelids. In the case of the upper one this can be done by taking hold of its central lashes, drawing it upward and outward, at the same time pressing its upper part downward, the patient meanwhile looking at his feet. The lower one can be everted by drawing it downward while the patient looks upward. The blood supply of the conjunctiva is derived mainly from the conjunctival arteries. They anastomose, around the cornea, with the muscular branches of the ciliary arteries and form the "peri-corneal zone." From this are given off vascular loops which penetrate the cornea to the depth of one millimetre.

The cornea is a beautifully transparent membrane forming the anterior sixth of the eyeball; it projects from the sclera in the form of a section of an ellipsoid; its radius of curvature is shorter than that of the sclera. The epithelium covering the anterior surface of the cornea is continuous with that of the conjunctiva, though modified, and it rests directly upon Bowman's membrane, which is a homogeneous layer consisting of a condensation of the cement substance of the next layer, which is called the true cornea or "substantia propria" or "stroma." It is made up of parallel laminae of white fibrous tissue; these are composed of bundles of fibers, and upon each bundle is found a fusiform nucleus. Chondrin-yielding cement substance holds the fibers and laminae together. Lymph spaces are found in the cement substance between the laminae; these are all connected and serve for the circulation of the lymph which nourishes the cornea. The blood-vessels extend into the corneal substance, forming loops which penetrate the substance of the cornea to the extent of one millimetre from its circumference towards its center. But few lymph cells are found in the lymph spaces during health. The true cornea is continuous with the sclera. The posterior limiting, or Descemet's, membrane is not so closely adherent to the true cornea as is Bowman's membrane. It is thin, strong and elastic and is covered with a single layer of endothelium. This membrane and its endothelium are continuous with the tissues of the iris. The nervous supply of the cornea is derived from the anterior ciliary and conjunctival nerves. Being richly supplied with nerves the cornea is exquisitely sensitive.

The iris and ciliary body form the anterior part of the uveal tract, being situated between the cornea and the ora serrata. Their stroma is continuous with that of the choroid, while the pigment layer which covers the inner surface of the ciliary body and the posterior surface of the iris is continuous with that of the retina. The epithelium covering the anterior surface of the iris and some of the elastic fibers found in its stroma are derived from Descemet's membrane of the cornea. The ciliary body is of an annular shape, about two-tenths of an inch wide, with a thick, round edge, directed anteriorly, and a thin edge, directed posteriorly, which is continuous with the choroid at the ora serrata. The ciliary body has a twofold function: first, to nourish the anterior part of the vitreous and crystalline lens and to secrete the aqueous humor; second, to perform the function of accommodation. For this reason it is divided into two parts: *(a)* the ciliary processes and folds, about seventy in number, and *(b)* the ciliary muscle, which consists of meridional, circular and radiating fibers. This muscle is the active agent in accommodation. The ciliary folds secrete the aqueous humor and nourish the lens and the anterior part of the vitreous. These folds are the most vascular part of the uveal tract; they are bound together by delicate connective tissue stroma, which contains numerous branched pigment cells. The inner surface of the ciliary body is covered by an elastic membrane, which is continuous with the laminae vitrea of the choroid. Upon this elastic membrane are two layers of cells derived from the retina; the cells of one layer are pigmented, those of the other non-pigmented; they are epithelial in character.

The iris is a membrane, circular in shape, with a central opening, called the pupil, whose function is to regulate the amount of light entering the eye; it does this by contracting and dilating the pupil. The stroma of the iris is made up, principally, of blood-vessels, which run in radiating directions. At a short distance from the pupil they give off branches and form a circle of vessels, which divides the iris into two zones — the pupillary zone, which surrounds the pupil, and the ciliary zone, which extends to the periphery of the iris. The blood-vessels are bound together by connective and elastic tissue containing connective tissue pigmented and non-pigmented cells. Within the stroma, near the pupillary margin and close to the posterior surface, are found circular fibers, whose function is to contract the pupil. As no radiating fibers have as yet been found in the iris of man, and as dilatation of the pupil is known to follow irritation of the sympathetic nerve, active dilatation is probably due to contraction of the blood-vessels, with which the iris is so abundantly supplied, passive dilatation being caused by contraction of the elastic membrane and fibers that are found in the iris. The tissue of the iris forms a very spongy membrane, and around the pupillary and ciliary circles numerous small spaces are found into which the epithelium dips. The iris and ciliary body are connected to the cornea and sclera by the ligamentum pectinatum, which is a mass of spongy tissue passing from the cornea and sclera to the iris and anterior part of the

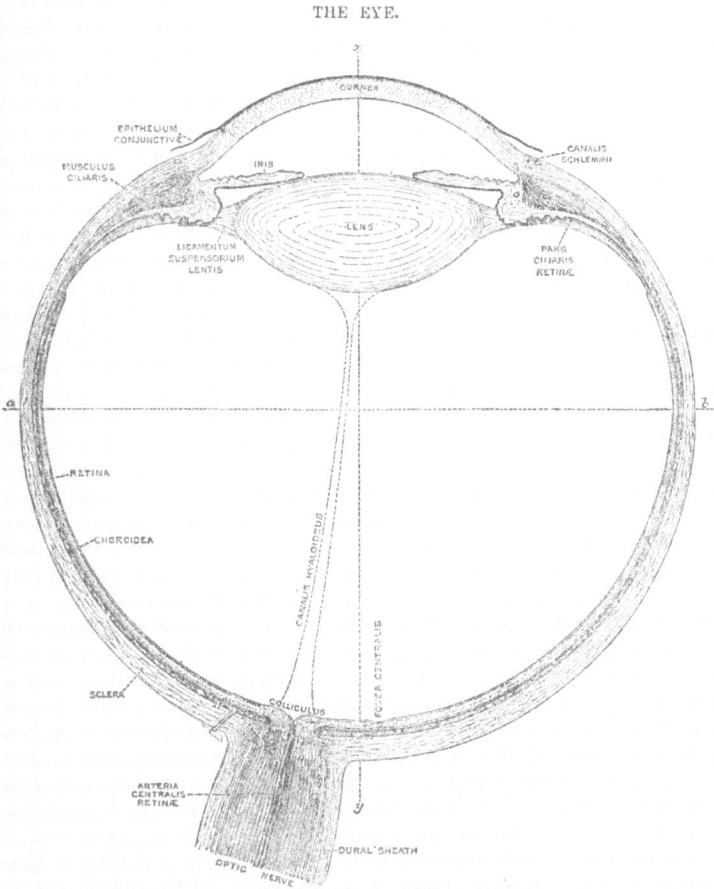

THE EYE.

ciliary body. The epithelium of Descemet's membrane passes between the bundles of fibers and supplies all this spongy tissue with an endothelial lining. This spongy tissue forms the inner surface of Schlemm's canal, a circular sinus lying near the corneoscleral junction. The fluids of the anterior part of the eye are supposed to escape through the loose tissue of the iritic angle into Schlemm's canal, and from that into the veins. The iris and ciliary body, with the lens capsule, the ligament of Zinn and the posterior surface of the cornea, form the boundaries of the aqueous chamber, the depth of which averages about 3 mm., though it is subject to great variation in health and disease. The iris divides this chamber into two parts, known as the anterior and posterior chambers. When the pupil is of average size the pupillary zone of the iris rests on the anterior capsule of the lens; it floats free in the aqueous humor when the pupil is dilated. The color of the iris depends upon the amount of pigment contained in its stroma, dark eyes having a large amount, blue eyes little or none. The nervous supply of the iris and ciliary body comes from the third, fifth and sympathetic nerves. The blood supply is from the anterior and long posterior ciliary arteries. Nearly all the blood is carried off by the vense vorticosae. The anterior ciliary veins which anastomose with the conjunctival veins carry off but a small amount of blood when the eye is free from disease.

The sclera is a dense white, fibrous membrane, extending from the cornea to the optic nerve entrance. It is about i mm. in thickness around the cornea and i.i mm. around the optic nerve entrance. It gives shape and support to the eyeball. All the ocular muscles are attached to it. A system of lymph canals, resembling those of the cornea, are found in this membrane. It is but scantily supplied with nerves. Its blood-vessels form a wide capillary network, and it is pierced by the nerves, arteries and veins that supply the intraocular tissues.

Chapter Two - Diseases of the Conjunctiva

Foreign bodies may lodge upon any part of the conjunctiva. If upon the conjunctival part of the lower lid or lower retrotarsal fold they may cause very little irritation, unless they are of a size or nature to interfere with the movements of the eyeball or to cause destruction of tissue. Very small particles on the inner surface of the lid or on the upper part of the ocular conjunctiva may cause only a sensation of roughness under the lids, or they may cause great pain with hyperaemia of the conjunctiva, lachrymation and spasmodic closure of the lids, and, if allowed to remain, a violent conjunctivitis may result. A careful examination of the conjunctiva should be made, a magnifying glass being used if necessary, first the lower then the upper lid being everted. If no foreign substance be found a 4% solution of Cocaine mur. should be dropped between the lids. A piece of absorbent cotton about the size of a pea should be wrapped upon a probe, and after being dipped into the solution of Cocaine it should be passed between the everted upper lid and the eyeball so as to carefully explore the upper fornix. This procedure will often bring out a foreign body that was hidden from sight. The cornea should also be carefully examined. Foreign bodies are best removed by means of a small piece of absorbent cotton or clean blotting paper. If adherent to the conjunctiva they may be removed by a gouge. If buried in the membrane, the foreign body with the adhering part of the conjunctiva should be lifted up with a small pair of fixation forceps and snipped off with a pair of curved, blunt-pointed scissors. For some time after a foreign body has been removed from an eye the patient may have the same sensations as before its removal. For the relief of these sensations a drop of Cocaine solution should be instilled between the eyelids. If the conjunctiva is congested give Aconite 2x, a tablet every hour; also direct the patient to bathe his eyelids every few minutes with cold water. In a short time this treatment will give relief.

Injuries to the Conjunctiva.

Lime, acids and molten metals splashed into the eye are the most frequent causes of injuries to the conjunctiva. The destruction of tissue may be very great, and not limited to the conjunctiva, but the cornea, sclera and even the whole eyeball may be destroyed. If the subconjunctival tissue is injured, healing will take place by the formation of a cicatrix, the contraction of which may cause distortion of the eyelids, interference with the passage of tears or limitations to the movements of the eyeball. If the epithelium of the neighboring parts of the palpebral and ocular conjunctiva or cornea are destroyed the lids may grow to the eyeball. Such a condition is called symblepharon. If the patient is seen soon after injury, the eye should be flooded with a bland oil and all the particles of foreign substance removed. Cocaine should be put into the eye to relieve the pain and permit of a thorough examination. Give Aeon, ix every hour. Put two drops of Almond oil in the eye every half hour, and bathe the eye frequently with cold water. If the burn has been an extensive one, symblepharon will probably form in spite of any treatment. (See Operation for Symblepharon.)

Wounds of the conjunctiva may be penetrating, cleancut or lacerated. They should be washed with a solution (.0001) of Merc, corr., and if they gap they should be sutured with sterilized iron-dyed silk. If this is not done granuloma may develop to the patient's great annoyance. If granuloma have formed do not attempt to remove them at once, but wait until their attachments become narrowed; then snip them off with scissors.

Ecchymosis.

Ecchymosis of the conjunctiva may result from blows on the head or eye, or it may be due to rupture of one of the conjunctival blood-vessels caused by violent coughing, sneezing or straining. It may occur during Bright's disease or scurvy, and it may be the forerunner of apoplexy. Hamamelis θ, a drop three times a day, seems to hasten absorption of the effusion.

Oedema.

Oedema of the conjunctiva is found as a symptom of inflammation; also in Bright's disease, in senile degeneration and in general debility. Apis mel. 3x is the remedy.

Emphysema.

Emphysema of the conjunctiva may be the result of rupture of the lachry-mal sac or of fracture of the nasal sinuses. A firm bandage should be applied to the eye.

Hyperaemia.

Hyperaemia of the conjunctiva may be the first symptom of a conjunctivi-tis, or it may be an essential condition. Of the latter form there are many causes, the most common being errors of refraction, accommodation or con-vergence I also diseases of the cornea, iris, ciliary body or orbit. It is very common in those persons who spend a large part of the time in foul, dusty or smoky places. The excessive use of stimulants, over-feeding, disease of the digestive organs, rheumatism and disease of the nose are frequently accom-panied by this trouble. Hyperaemia of the conjunctiva may be acute or chron-ic; if acute, the vascularity of both the palpebral and ocular conjunctiva will be greater than normal, the flow of tears and mucus will be increased, the conjunctiva will be swollen, and the patient will complain of a rough burning sensation with the feeling as of a foreign body under the eyelids, and general-ly of a lack of ability to use the eyes for any length of time, more especially by artificial light. In the chronic form the symptoms are the same, though less in degree, and the ocular conjunctiva, as a rule, is not affected. The pathological changes seem to be a dilatation of the blood-vessels, with an abnormal change in the amount of secretion of the mucous and lachrymal glands but no abnormal increase of tissue change. The treatment must depend upon the cause. Any existing refractive or muscular error must be corrected with great care. (See Errors of Refraction.) The eye symptoms are not sufficiently char-acteristic for the prescription of remedies. Consult Nux vomica, Belladonna, Ipecac, Arsenicum, Rhus tox , and Sulphur. Bathing the eyes with hot water will often give great relief.

CONJUNCTIVITIS.

(INFLAMMATION OF THE CONJUNCTIVA.)

Superficial conjunctivitis may be divided into simple and toxic. Some of the synonyms for these forms are catarrhal, muco-purulent, epidemic and

14

autumnal conjunctivitis. Slight redness of the palpebral conjunctiva, a watery discharge and a tendency of the lids to stick together may be the only symptoms in mild cases of superficial conjunctivitis. In the severe cases other symptoms are added, such as photophobia, lachrymation, a mucous discharge, oedema of the ocular conjunctiva, swelling of the eyelids, Small hemorrhages in the conjunctiva, a feeling as of sand in the eyes and pain in and around the eyes. The disease may be acute or chronic, and may last from a few hours to many months. The pathological changes of this form of conjunctivitis are dilatation of the blood-vessels, stasis of the circulating blood, exudation of corpuscles and of lymph which contains all the elements for the formation of fibrin. These are the changes which cause most of the swelling found in this trouble. In addition to the vascular changes, the epithelial cells rapidly proliferate and are cast off in an immature condition. These imperfectly developed epithelial cells, together with some wandering cells form the cellular part of the secretion. The death of some of these elements cause the discharge to become muco-purulent. The mucous glands are filled with and secrete a larger quantity of mucus than under normal conditions. The inflamed membrane regains its normal state by its vessels regaining their tone, by the cessation of exudation and the absorption of the remaining exudates, by the epithelia maturing and the secretion of the mucous glands becoming normal. The toxic forms of this trouble are without doubt due to micro-organism, and as a consequence they are contagious. As there is no way of distinguishing the toxic forms from the simple forms — except by a bacteriological examination — the physician will do well to treat all forms as if they were contagious, and to warn the patient and those about him of the danger they are in if they do not observe proper care and cleanliness. To destroy and remove the bacilli and free the eye of irritating secretions that tend to keep up inflammatory conditions, a non-irritating disinfectant should be freely used as an eye-wash; this will not only put the patient in a condition to recover, but will tend to prevent the spread cf the disease to others; and, if only one eye is affected, rigid cleanliness may prevent the disease from spreading to the other eye. But it should be clearly understood that these measures will not take the place of the homoeopathic remedies unless • the solution happens to contain the indicated remedy. It requires something more than bacilli to set up a conjunctivitis; for one thing the tissues must be in a condition to nourish the bacilli or they will die. It is to remedy this state of the tissues and to remove the conditions remaining after the cause of the inflammation has been removed, that internal medication is used. Among the remedies found to be of most value are Aconite for the first stages, when the hyperaemia is great and the discharge slight, especially if the patient is intolerant of pain; it is frequently indicated in traumatic conjunctivitis, to be given in first decimal and the dose frequently repeated. Apis when there is a marked oedema of the conjunctiva and eyelids, the oedematous swelling of the ocular conjunctiva having a translucent appearance, first or third decimal in frequent doses. Ant. tart, in the chronic forms with a tendency to thickening of the membrane and obstruction of the ducts of the tarsal glands, to be given not lower than the third decimal, morning and night. Arnica in the traumatic forms where the hyperaemia is not great but the feeling of soreness is marked, third decimal, a dose every hour. Arsenicum for both the acute and chronic forms when the discharge is free and watery with a tendency to excoriate the skin of the face, burning pain, a feeling of soreness when moving the eyeballs, photophobia and twitching of the eyelids, to be given three times a day not lower than the third decimal or higher than the sixth. Aurum muriaticum when the conjunctivitis is chronic with follicular enlargements, the third decimal, given three times a day. Belladonna in both the acute and chronic forms when the conjunctiva looks red and the eyes feel very dry and hot, with swelling of the eyelids and a flickering of light before the eyes, first or third decimal, a dose every two hours. Euphrasia ix in the mild muco-purulent forms with a free discharge somewhat acrid in character, with a tendency of the mucus to adhere to the cornea and accumulate in the corners of the eyelids, dose to be repeated hourly. Ipecac in the subacute forms when the conjunctiva is swollen and not very red, and when the discharge is almost pure mucus, third decimal, three times a day. Merc. sol. in both acute and chronic forms, with itching of the eyes and a muco-purulent excoriating discharge, and a feeling as though the eyelids were stuck to the eyeball, marked dread of artificial light, third to the sixth decimal, three times a day. Puis, in acute and chronic conditions, discharge thick, yellow and bland, with puffy eyelids and a tendency of the discharge to spread all over the eyeball, first decimal, three times a day. Sulphur in the chronic forms which show a tendency to relapse, with sticking pains worse in the morning, third or sixth decimal, once a day. The best disinfectant for the eye-wash seems to be a .0001 solution of Merc. corr. in distilled water. In severe cases the eyes should be washed every hour by freely dropping this solution into the conjunctival sac and wiping away the secretion with absorbent cotton, which should be immediately burnt after being used. Neither bandages, poultices, wet or dry rags, nor anything that tends to retain the secretion within the eyelids should be tolerated, for all such things have a tendency to convert slight cases into severe ones. A small quantity of bland oil may be spread on the edge of the eyelids at night to keep them from sticking together. The cornea and iris should be examined during the course of superficial conjunctivitis, for inflammation of the cornea and iris sometimes accompany this condition.

PURULENT CONJUNCTIVITIS

(PURULENT INFLAMMATION OF THE CONJUNCTIVA.)

The most characteristic picture of purulent conjunctivitis is presented in the gonorrheal form, as seen in the adult. There is scarcely a doubt that this form is caused by direct contact with gonorrheal secretion, as gonococci have been repeatedly found in its secretion. Pure cultures of the bacilli found in gonorrheal secretion and placed on the conjunctiva have set up purulent conjunctivitis. The bacilli may be conveyed to the eye from the sexual organs or from an eye suffering from purulent conjunctivitis, generally by the fingers or by towels that have been used by persons suffering from gonorrhea or gonorrheal conjunctivitis. In opening the eyes of a person suffering from this disease great care must be used, as the secretion may spurt from the palpebral opening with great force and for a considerable distance. Many eyes have been lost in this way, for the disease thus set up is generally violent.

The eyelids should be separated by slowly drawing down the lower lid to allow the secretion to escape and then lifting the upper one. Fresh air, sunlight, dilution and drying tend to destroy the infective power of the secretion. If the disease is to be very intense the first symptoms will be manifest in a few hours from the time of the infection; the milder forms may not show any marked symptoms for three days. In the first stage of a severe case the eyelids are red, hot and swollen to such an extent that it is very difficult to open them. The palpebral conjunctiva and the retrotarsal folds are intensely hyperaemic and greatly swollen; the ocular conjunctiva is also red and swollen to such an extent that the cornea is often lost to view. This swelling of the ocular conjunctiva is called chemosis. The eyelids are sensitive and feel hard to the touch. In places the conjunctiva may appear of a grayish-yellow color, or a whitish membrane may cover its surface. The discharge at this stage is thin, watery and of a reddish-yellow tint. In the second stage the swelling grows less, the eyelids wrinkle and the discharge becomes free and seems to consist entirely of pus. The lymphatic glands in front of the ear may be swollen, and the patient's temperature is apt to be increased. Resolution may take place at the end of this stage or the disease may pass into a third stage, called the chronic form, which is characterized by a thickening and velvety appearance of the palpebral conjunctiva and scant} discharge from the eye. In a mild case the symptoms may be those of a muco-purulent conjunctivitis and only distinguished from it by an examination of the micro-organisms contained in the discharge. The pathological changes in purulent conjunctivitis differ from those found in catarrhal inflammation in that the inflammatory changes involve the deeper tissues of the conjunctiva and the inflammatory lymph exuded into the conjunctival and subconjunctival tissues tend to coagulate within as well as on the surface of the conjunctiva. The greatest danger of this disease — the destruction of the cornea — is attributed to these changes, as well as to the infective nature of the discharge and the marked tendency to death of the cellular elements and consequent rapid formation of pus. The exudation within the conjunctiva is sometimes so great as to cut off all nutrition from the cornea, so it dies from necrosis, the whole membrane sloughing away with the exception of a narrow rim around its circumference;

if this takes place the iris and ciliary body will become involved in the destructive changes; panophthalmitis may result, leaving in place of the eye a more than worthless stump, which may in time set up sympathetic inflammation in the other eye. If the cornea escapes the dangers of this stage, it may suffer from various forms of ulceration at a later stage.

The most dangerous of these is the circular ulcer that forms around the circumference of the cornea, sometimes causing destruction of this membrane. Small or large ulcers may form on any part of the cornea. The later in the course of the disease that ulceration of the cornea appears the more chance there will be of limiting its extent and the more favorable will be the prognosis. The course of the disease may extend from a few days to many weeks, depending upon its severity and the treatment adopted. The first step in the treatment is to put the patient to bed, and if only one eye is inflamed to protect the other one; this can be done by placing a watch crystal over the sound eye, holding it in place by a piece of rubber plaster from which a hole has been cut, leaving the center of the glass uncovered so that the patient can see through it and to also allow the attendant to inspect the eye. The piaster should be made to adhere closely to the face, except at the lower edge, where a small opening should be left to allow the tears to find an outlet. The patient must not be allowed to sleep on the side that contains the sound eye. Two nurses should be employed, one to serve all night and the other to serve all day. They should wash and remove all secretion from the eye every fifteen minutes. For this wash a .0001 solution of Merc. corr. should be used in the first stage of the disease. A quantity of this solution should be put into a large vessel containing a large piece of ice. Small pieces of cotton cloth that have been cooled on this ice should be placed on the eyelids and changed as often as they become warm; at the same time they must not be used to reduce the temperature of the lids below the normal on account of the danger of depriving the cornea of its nutrition. No strong or irritating solutions should be used at this stage, but the eye must be kept free from any accumulation of its secretion. If the swelling of the eyelids is so great that they can not be opened, the outer canthus should be cut through with a pair of strong scissors; this will allow the eyelids to open and it will also relieve the cornea of a great amount of pressure. It is only in severe cases that this operation is necessary. Veratrum vir. 1x, a dose every half hour, is an excellent remedy in this stage. The second stage, that of purulent discharge, demands incessant cleanliness and the application of a 2% solution of Argent, nit. to the palpebral conjunctiva, especially along the retrotarsal folds. This application is best made by means of a earners hair brush. Allow the solution to remain on the conjunctiva until a white film forms on the surface of the membrane, then wash oil with plenty of pure water. Ulceration is not a counter-indication to the use of Argent, nit., but none of the solution should be allowed to touch the cornea, especially the ulcerated spot. The lids should be everted before applying the solution, and it should be washed off before they are returned to their normal position. The application should be made once in every twenty-four hours until the discharge ceases. Clinical experience has shown that Argent, nit. is superior to any other germicide in this affection, but it must not be used in the first stage. Puls, is the remedy most frequently indicated in the first stage; first decimal, three times a day. For the chronic form use a .0001 solution of Merc, corr., two drops in the eye every morning, and give Antimonium tart. 3x, three times a day. It must be borne well in mind that this disease is very contagious. The mild forms of gonorrheal ophthalmia should be treated as muco-purulent conjunctivitis.

Ophthalmia Neonatorum.

Ophthalmia neonatorum is a form of purulent conjunctivitis that occurs in the new-born. It is generally due to contagion at the time of birth, either from a gonorrheal or an acrid leucorrheal discharge. The secretion taken from a large number of cases have shown the gonococci. The disease generally shows itself on the second or third day; if it appears later than the fifth day, the assumption is that the eye was inoculated after birth. As a rule, it runs a milder course than purulent conjunctivitis in the adult; but it is a very destructive disease, being one of the greatest causes of blindness. The treatment should be the same as for a case of purulent conjunctivitis in the adult, with the exception of the cold applications, which the infant does not bear well. The solution of Merc, com should be used at least every half hour day and night. In the second stage the 2% solution of Argent, nit. should be used once in every four hours. The mother and attendants should be warned of the serious nature of the disease and of the danger of infection to themselves and others. As a prophylactic the vagina of the pregnant woman may be washed out, just before birth takes place, with a .0001 solution of Merc. corr. A drop of a 2% solution of Argent. nit. may be put into each eye of the child immediately after birth.

Hepar sulph. 3x, a tablet every morning, and evening when the secretion of pus is very free, is, in my opinion the best remedy. If the secretion is scanty, give Aconite. Purulent conjunctivitis not due to gonorrhea sometimes occurs in persons of depraved constitutions. Calc. hypophos. 1x, a grain three times a day, is indicated in this condition.

CIRCUMSCRIBED CONJUNCTIVITIS.

(CIRCUMSCRIBED INFLAMMATION OF THE CONJUNCTIVA.)

Circumscribed conjunctivitis may present several forms, but their etiology, clinical history and treatment are so much alike that they may be considered under one head. The typical form of phlyctenular conjunctivitis first manifests itself by the appearance of one or more cone-shaped, pale reddish-yellow elevations of the epithelium of the conjunctiva at or near the limbus.

These may vary in diameter from 1 to 3 mm. If only one phlyctenule is present it is generally larger than when there are several, and the hyperemia of the conjunctiva is confined to a triangular area, the apex of which is situated at the base of the phlyctenule, its base being lost in the conjunctiva. When there are a large number of phlyctenules present at one time the redness of the conjunctiva may be general. Lachrymation is a prominent symptom, and photophobia is sometimes present. Spasm of the eyelids (blepharospasm) is often an annoying symptom. The lachrymation sometimes causes a dermatitis of the eyelids and face. A phlyctenule may go through all its stages in from eight to fourteen days. There is great tendency to relapse, new phlyctenules sometimes appearing before the old ones have disappeared, and then again after many months. This disease is rarely limited to the conjunctiva, the cornea being very apt to become involved. (See Disease of the Cornea.) Catarrhal or muco-purulent conjunctivitis may complicate this disease. The pathological changes are an aggregation of cellular elements around a terminal nerve fiber. This exudation takes place in the tissues of the conjunctiva, and is the cause of the cone-shaped elevations of its epithelium. As the disease progresses the epithelium over the apex of the cone breaks down, leaving an ulcer with base and edges raised above the general level of the conjunctiva. The death and elimination of the exudated cellular elements leaves a superficial ulceration of the conjunctiva, which is soon covered by epithelia and generally leaves no visible cicatrix. The pustular form is manifested by the formation of pus within the exudation. The pus escapes, leaving an ulcerated surface, which runs the same course as phlyctenular ulceration. The vesicular form generally appears on the palpebral portion of the conjunctiva, appearing as several small elevations of its epithelium; these contain a clear fluid; they break and leave small ulcers which soon heal. All these forms of circumscribed conjunctivitis are very common, especially among poorly nourished children. The great danger is the involvement of the cornea. (See Diseases of the Cornea.) As all these forms are markedly constitutional the main reliance in treatment must be internal medication. Among the remedies most frequently indicated are Pulsatilla, Calc. phos., Merc, dulc, Merc, corr., Heparsulph., Arsen. In prescribing, the general symptoms will have to be the guide. The patient should receive good nourishing food, salt water baths three times a week, and he should spend a large part of the time in the open air. No bandage is to be worn, but he may wear light smoke-colored glasses. Warn the patient that the disease is apt to become chronic, and of the necessity of continuing the treatment for some time.

PLASTIC CONJUNCTIVITIS

(PLASTIC INFLAMMATION OF THE CONJUNCTIVA.)

The form of inflammation of the conjunctiva termed diphtheritic is due to infection by the bacillus diphtherias, and is generally characterized by swelling and great hardness of the eyelids, a reddened conjunctiva interspaced with grayish-white spots, which seem to be depressed below the level of the general surface of the conjunctiva. Sometimes these coalesce and the whole conjunctiva appears like a piece of dirty-gray shrunken leather. The conjunctiva may be covered with a closely adherent grayish-white membrane. A thin acrid discharge appears in the early stages; at a later period the membrane is undermined and thrown off, and the discharge becomes purulent. The pathological changes are generally an exudation and coagulation of fibrinous material in and upon the conjunctiva, though in some of the most malignant cases no membrane forms, the exudation seeming to be wholly within the tissues; it often results in the destruction and slouching of the affected part of the conjunctiva. The lost tissue is replaced by granulation; healing is completed by the formation of a cicatrix, the subsequent contraction of which may cause distortion of the eyelids, resulting in entropion, trichiasis, etc. If opposite portions of the ocular and palpebral conjunctiva slough, symplepharon will probably result. Great care must be used in cleansing the eye, as the slightest abrasion of the cornea will allow the diphtheritic membrane to form there. Partial or complete destruction of the cornea is almost certain to occur, either by extension of the disease to it, or by ulceration, or by a necrosis clue to lack of nutrition. It is a very rare disease in this country. Its treatment must be that of diphtheria, of which it may be only a local manifestation.

Merc. cyan. 3x is the remedy that has given me the most satisfaction, supplemented by a very mild antiseptic solution to keep the eye clean. Irritants are decidedly contra-indicated. Cold applications, while they check the growth of the bacilli, should not be used to any extent because they interfere with the nourishment of the cornea. Croupous conjunctivitis is said to exist when an easily removable membrane forms on the conjunctiva. Its removal leaves a more or less raw surface. The swelling of the eyelids is soft. The disease runs a chronic course, the membrane reforming many times. It is of very rare occurrence and seldom involves the cornea. Iodine 6x is the remedy, a tablet three times a day. In several diseases of the conjunctiva, such as purulent, traumatic and phlyctenular conjunctivitis, false membranes may form on the conjunctiva. Burns from lime, or Argent, nit. or inflammation due to the use of jequirity, present marked appearances of croupous or diphtheritic conjunctivitis, and might be mistaken for either of them if the history of the case was not inquired into. The diagnosis of diphtheritic conjunctivitis can be conclusively made by a microscopic examination and inoculation of another mucous membrane.

GRANULAR CONJUNCTIVITIS. FOLLICULAR CONJUNCTIVITIS.

Granular conjunctivitis has numerous synonyms, as trachoma, trachomatous conjunctivitis, blenorrhoea, Egyptian or military ophthalmia, etc., etc. Trachoma is probably the least misleading of any of these names. There is no doubt but that this disease is contagious, and that it becomes violently so when a large number of persons are huddled together under unsanitary conditions, poverty and dirt being the predisposing causes. It is a very common disease in orphan asylums, poorhouses and barracks. Fresh air, good food and personal cleanliness exert great power in destroying its contagious property. Physicians and others who handle diseased eyes should be very careful to wash their hands with some disinfecting solution after examining one eye and before examining another. Sattler and Michel have isolated a diplococcus which differs from the gonococcus, in that it is smaller and its line of division is not so well marked, while gelatine is not liquified by it and Gram's process does not deprive it of its color. Inoculation of the healthy human conjunctiva by this diplococcus, or "trachococcus," has produced granular conjunctivitis. Trachoma is a disease which presents very different symptoms in its various stages. At one stage the patient may complain only of a slight weakness of the eyes, with a disagreeable feeling in the morning. Inspection of the conjunctiva may show numerous translucent, grayish yellow, hemispherical bodies about the size of a small pin's head, which push up the surface of the conjunctiva. These may be found scattered along the retrotarsal folds and along the convex border of the tarsal cartilage of the upper lid, the conjunctiva not being redder than normal and the secretion being very slightly greater than in health. In other cases the granular bodies may cover the entire palpebral, and extend to the ocular, conjunctiva, or even to the conjunctival layer of the cornea. The granules may have lost their translucent appearance and present a bright red hue, the whole conjunctiva looking like a mass of granulation tissue, photophobia, lachrymation and a scanty muco-purulent discharge being present. In other cases the normal folds or papilke of the conjunctiva become greatly enlarged and hide the granules from view, the whole conjunctiva looking like a piece of coarse red velvet, the retrotarsal folds rolling out like fleshy masses when the lids are everted. Again the appearance may be as of granules and papillae mixed together; this form is very common. The cases that present the marked papillary enlargement are often mistaken for the chronic stage of purulent conjunctivitis, and vice versa. During the course of any of these cases, or even before any sign of trachoma has become manifest, a violent inflammation of the conjunctiva, which may include the cornea, may set in, the lids appearing heavy and swollen, the conjunctiva very red, greatly swollen, smooth and glistening, all signs of the papillae or granulations being lost. Severe pain and photophobia are marked symptoms. The cornea may be covered by pannus or by ulcers that show a marked tendency to perforate. An eye which has been destroyed by trachoma might be mistaken for one that had been severely burned by lime or by a strong acid. The pathological changes of this disease differ from those of catarrhal, purulent and diphtheritic conjunctivitis, in that the primary changes are in the lymphoid and fibrous tissue elements, the vascular and epithelial changes seeming to be secondary. The reason trachoma is such a very mild disease in some cases and in others so very destructive is probably due to the condition of the system when inoculation takes place, and also to the amount and virulence of the inoculating material. In the very mild cases the pathological changes are limited to an aggregation of lymphoid elements and a consequent enlargement of the lymphatic follicles, with proliferation of a few connective tissue cells and the formation of a slight amount of cicatricial tissue. As the disease progresses some of the lymphoid cells break down and are absorbed; the breaking down of these cells gives the follicles the yellowish color they sometimes present. The scar tissue shows itself by a few narrow" white bands. In the mild cases these scars are very few and run in a direction parallel with the free margin of the lids. No perceptible change in the function of the eye can be noticed. As the disease progresses in severity the granules, which consist of an aggregation of lymphoid cells and of proliferating connective tissue corpuscles, increase in number and may be found in all parts of the palpebral, ocular and corneal conjunctiva. In addition there may be inflammatory changes in other tissues of the conjunctiva or cornea. At any stage of granular conjunctivitis the pathological conditions of a severe muco-purulent inflammation may be added to the changes proper to trachoma. The changes that occur in the cornea are a proliferation and extension of the blood-vessels from the marginal to the transparent portion ^of the cornea; these vessels are generally found in the superficial layers. In addition to the vascular changes proliferating, spindle shaped cells are found, especially under Bowman's membrane. The conditions that result from these changes in the cornea are called pannus. It generally occurs at the upper part of the cornea first, but may extend to any part of it. The roughness of the lids is supposed to favor its development at this point, yet they cannot be the only factor, because pannus occurs at the upper part of the cornea when the lid is smooth. Its starting point is generally at the limbus and is probably due to a deposit of contagious material at this point, although it may be a direct extension of the inflammatory changes from the ocular conjunctiva. The essential pathological factor in granular conjunctivitis is the proliferation of the connective tissue elements and the formation of the young cicatricial tissue not only in the conjunctival membrane, but within the subconjunctival tissue, the tarsal cartilages and even in the cornea. It is this formation that distinguishes trachoma from all other forms of conjunctival inflammation. The loss of function and subsequent degeneration of the conjunctiva and the eye are due, primarily, to the contraction of this new tissue; it causes the obliteration and destruction of the conjunctival glands and the obliteration of the ducts of the lachrymal and Meibomian glands, the distortion of the tarsal cartilage and consequent entropion, trichiasis, distichiasis, shrinking of the conjunctiva and fatty degeneration of its epithelium with a resultant xerosis. Trachoma generally runs a very chronic course, with periods of marked remission and exacerbation. Recovery may take place at any stage of the disease, and the functional condition of the eye will depend upon the amount of destructive change that has taken place. Recent superficial pannus may disappear and leave the cornea clear and transparent. If the pannus has continued for a long time, or if ulceration of the cornea has occurred, a clear cornea cannot be expected. If xerosis results very little can be done. In the treatment of trachoma one thing must be borne in mind — that is, that strong caustics or destructive agents of any kind must never be used. In cases where pannus is very dense, eyes have been inoculated with gonorrheal pus and jequirity has also been used to clear up the pannus; and, while in some cases these measures have seemed to clear the cornea, they are very dangerous agents to use. A solution of Merc, corr., containing one-tenth of a grain to the ounce of distilled water, should be freely used in all stages of this disease, three or four drops to be placed within the eyelids three times a day. This solution serves to disinfect the discharge and so prevent the spread of the disease; it also serves to check the growth of the bacilli within the conjunctiva, and so removes the cause of the trouble.

Aurum mur. 3x is the medicine most frequently indicated in all stages of this disease; it seems to have the power of checking the formation of the fibrous tissue; it is to be given three times a day. Daring the inflammatory exacerbations, Aurum may be discontinued for a time and Apis mel. Θ given if the swelling of the eyelids is very great. If the swelling is not so marked, but the redness and pain intense, Aeon, ix should be given every half hour; at the same time cloths wet in a cold solution of Merc, corr. should be laid on the eyelids and changed as soon as they become warm. Surgical measures that destroy the integrity of the conjunctiva are not to be recommended.

Follicular Conjunctivitis.

Enlarged follicles frequently appear in the retrotarsal folds of the eyes of children and delicate adults, also from the application of solutions of Atropine and Eserine in the cases of persons who are very susceptible to these poisons. The follicles appear as pale, translucent, gray bodies, oval in shape and situated beneath the conjunctiva. They bear a very close resemblance to trachomatous granules, and sometimes can only be distinguished from them by their location and by the different pathological changes that take place in the two conditions. The follicles are never situated on the cartilage of the upper lid, and cicatricial changes never take place in them. After remaining for a longer or shorter period they disappear. Sometimes attacks of inflammation of the conjunctiva accompany the follicles and obscure the condition. A diagnosis should not be attempted at this stage; simply treat the inflammation. Follicular conjunctivitis may be complicated with trachoma. In such cases the disease should be called trachoma and be treated as such. Fresh air is the best remedy. Among the medicines that may be of value are Calc. phos., Puis., Hepar sulph., Calc. iod., and Arsenicum. If in doubt as to diagnosis treat it as a mild case of trachoma.

ULCERS, TUMORS, HYPERTROPHY, ATROPHY, AND DEGENERATION OF THE CONJUNCTIVA, VERNAL AND EXANTHEMATOUS CONJUNCTIVITIS.

Vernal Conjunctivitis.

Vernal conjunctivitis — so called by Saemish, who first described it — is a very rare disease. It occurs in the spring and early summer, disappears in the winter and recurs again the following spring, and so on for several years. It is generally accompanied by other symptoms of chronic catarrh. It is found mostly in children and young adults. The pathological changes are described as consisting of an accumulation of conjunctival epithelial cells, more especially at the limbus, looking like a smooth, pale, yellowish-gray mound. The conjunctiva is infiltrated and the enlarged papillae are flattened and look like paving stones. It generally attacks both eyes and may clear up perfectly. Treatment does not seem to have been very satisfactory, but we have no record of any case being treated by a homeopathic physician.

Exanthematous Conjunctivitis.

Conjunctivitis that occurs during the course of measles, smallpox, scarlet fever, acne rosacea, etc., may assume any of the forms of inflammation of the conjunctiva. The treatment must vary with the form of the trouble.

Ulcers of the Conjunctiva.

The most destructive ulceration of the conjunctiva is the tubercular form or lupus of the conjunctiva, as it is sometimes called. It may start in any part of the conjunctiva and run a very slow and most generally a painless course. It presents an ulcerated surface, with raised and nodular edges. It is exceedingly destructive, both eyelids and eyeball may be lost. The diagnosis is established by finding the tubercular bacillus. The treatment is thorough removal of the diseased tissue and cauterization of the cavity by the galvano-cautery. Ulcers of the conjunctiva may be due to conjunctivitis, to chalazion, to traumatism and to epithelioma. Syphilitic ulcers are very rare, and when found are most frequently near the edge of the lids. The treatment of ulcers of the conjunctiva will depend upon the cause.

Pterygium — True and False.

True pterygium may be divided into progressive and non-progressive. It is found only at the outer and inner sides of the cornea, and is a triangular fold of the conjunctiva. Its apex, which is a mass of degenerated conjunctival tissue, is firmly adherent to the cornea. Its base is lost in the conjunctiva, which is so tightly drawn that it is thrown into folds, and at its neck — the part that connects the base with the apex — a probe can be passed beneath the fold for some distance but never completely under the pterygium. The pathological changes in the pterygium are the same as those of Pinguecula. Histologically, they consist of an increase of elastic fibers and a deposit of colloid substance. When these changes invade the limbus of the cornea the conjunctiva becomes adherent to it, and in some cases the degeneration extends across the cornea. As it encroaches on the pupillary space it limits the sight, and may cause complete blindness by covering the pupil. The progressive forms may be distinguished from the non-progressive by their thick, soft and vascular appearance, the stationary form appearing pale and thin. Pseudo-pterygium may occur at any part of the cornea, and is generally due to the conjunctiva of the eyeball becoming adherent to an ulcerated or abraded surface of the cornea. It may resemble the true pterygium, but a probe can generally be passed under its neck. If either form is progressing, or is large enough to interfere with the movements of the eye, or if they cause annoyance, they should be removed by operation. (See Operations.)

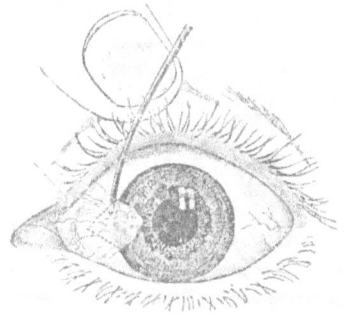

Pterygium.

Xerosis.

Xerosis may be primary or secondary, partial or complete. The partial form may accompany hemeralopia and may consist of one or two spots, which are not moistened by tears. The complete form generally occurs with some grave illness, and is frequently associated with keratomalacia. The pathological changes seem to be fatty degeneration of the epithelium of the conjunctiva, and sometimes of the lachrymal glands. The secondary form follows trachoma, diphtheria, pemphigus, burns of the conjunctiva, etc. It sometimes occurs in lagophthalmus induced by the constant exposure of the eyeball. This form can be relieved by an operation. The other forms are incurable in our present state of knowledge.

Tumors of the Conjunctiva.

Tumors that affect other mucous membranes may occur in the conjunctiva. The treatment is prompt removal.

Degenerations of the Conjunctiva.

Amyloid degeneration of the conjunctiva is a very rare condition. It appears as a chronic translucent swelling. There is no pain. Its chemical reaction is that of amyloid material.

Calcification of the Conjunctiva.

This occurs in small spots, and may be removed by means of a gouge.

Chapter Three - Diseases of The Cornea

The healthy cornea is a beautifully transparent membrane, and, being the principal refracting surface of the eye, all rays of light that go to form the ocular image must go through it. Consequently the slightest deviation from its normal transparency, or any alteration of curvature in its pupillary area, will impair vision. Nearly all diseases of the cornea manifest themselves either by a change of transparency or of curvature.

Examination of the Cornea.

An examination of the cornea is best made by oblique illumination, and preferably by artificial light. The method is as follows: a convex lens of about three-inch focus and of an inch and a half diameter is held between the index finger and thumb of the examiner, at about one foot from the lamp, which should be placed at one side of the patient's head. This lens will cause the rays of light to converge, and they should be thrown obliquely upon the cornea, the position of the lens being made to vary so that all parts of the cornea are successively illuminated, the relative positions of the patient and the light being also changed so that the illumination will come first from one side and then from the other, then from above, then from below. This examination will often show minute foreign bodies or opacities that were not visible by diffuse light. The normal cornea should be studied as regards its transparency, curvature and polish. The cornea of the young is very bright and reflects external objects, like a highly polished convex mirror. As life advances it loses its brilliancy and becomes less transparent. In the cornea of middle aged and old persons arcs of grayish opacity (called Areus senilis or Gerontoxon) appear; first at the upper, then at the lower, part; these arcs often join and form a circle, which is sharply separated from the limbus by a ring of transparent cornea. Arcus senilis is due to colloid degeneration; it is of very little importance and can be easily distinguished from ulceration by the corneal epithelium remaining intact. It is situated too far outside of the pupillary area to interfere with vision, nor do wounds in it fail to heal.

Foreign Bodies.

Foreign substances in or on the cornea may give rise to very slight or very severe symptoms. If the foreign body simply rests upon the cornea, and has not been there for any length of time, the patient may not be aware of its presence. If it was driven against the cornea with great force, or has been rubbed into the cornea by the patient in his vain attempts to remove it, or if it were hot or of a rough or acrid nature, the symptoms may resemble those of a sharp attack of iritis or keratitis, such as lachrymation, photophobia, severe pain, ciliary injection, hyperaemia of the conjunctiva, etc. To remove foreign bodies a 4% solution of Cocaine is to be dropped upon the cornea, and as soon as the tissues become insensible direct the patient to seat himself upon a firm chair and remove his hat. Then put a towel over his head, stand behind him and let his head rest against your breast; then direct him to open both his eyes and turn them so as to bring the foreign body into view. Hold the eye open by pressing the eyelids apart with the thumb and index finger of the left hand, at the same time making gentle pressure on the eyeball, thus serving to fix it. Most foreign bodies can thus be best removed by a piece of absorbent cotton, wrapped around a probe, with which the foreign body can be gently rubbed from the cornea. This method should be tried in all cases, unless the substance is deeply imbedded in the cornea. In the last named case a spud may be used by placing it under the foreign body and gently lifting it, being very careful all the while not to allow the spud to slip and scrape the cornea, or to press with such force as to perforate it. A pair of fine forceps is best to remove large foreign bodies that have penetrated deeply into the cornea. Foreign bodies, if not removed, set up an ulceration of the cornea surrounding them, and they may be thrown off in this way. The impairment of sight resulting from a foreign body will depend upon the location and amount of destruction of tissue, caused by its presence or by the efforts at removal. A very minute scar in the center of the cornea will cause great impairment of sight, while a very large one near the limbus may cause very little, if any. The healing of the wound in the cornea is generally rapid, although in old or worn-out subjects a small injury by a foreign body may be the starting-point of a destructive inflammation. Wounds and injuries of the cornea are to be treated by cleansing the eye with a mild antiseptic solution, and applying a bandage to protect and keep the eye at rest. If the injury is near the center of the cornea, the pupil should be dilated by a mydriatic. If near the limbus, a myotic to contract the pupil should be used, providing the iris has not been injured. When traumatic keratitis is very severe, the iris frequently participates in the inflammation, and in such a case the pupil should be kept widely dilated. Patients should be warned that even a slight injury, if near the center of the cornea, may seriously impair vision. Cold applications are best in the early stages of traumatic inflammation of the cornea. Acon, 1x is the remedy when the pains are very severe, the conjunctiva being of a bright red color with little swelling. Hepar sulph. 3x when the eye throbs and is very sensitive to touch, and when a grayish-yellow haze surrounds the site of injury threatening suppuration, or if suppuration has already taken place, it is still more strongly indicated. Rhus tox. 3x when the oedema of the conjunctiva and swelling of the lids are marked, the conjunctiva being of a dusky red, pain of an aching character, suppuration seeming imminent. Calc. hypophos. ix in old wornout subjects and in children suffering from malnutrition. Such patients are best kept in bed with the eye bandaged, the eye being kept clean, the bandage frequently changed and the patient's nutrition being kept up by good food and hygienic surroundings.

Inflammations and Degenerations of the Cornea

The cornea being anatomically continuous with the conjunctiva, iris, ciliary body and sclera, any inflammation of these structures is apt to spread to it. Forming a part of the external envelop of the eyeball, the structure and shape of the cornea influences and is influenced by the intraocular tension. Diseases of the cornea may be divided into those that cause destruction of the corneal tissue, and those that cause only opacities or deviations from its normal curvature. Phlyctenular keratitis, abscess and ulcers, vesicular keratitis and keratitis bulbosa are types of disease that cause marked destruction of the corneal tissue.

Phlyctenular Keratitis.

Synonyms: Lymphatic, pustular, scrofulous, marginal, etc.
It is the most common of all the diseases of the cornea. Like phlyctenular conjunctivitis it is found frequently in poorly nourished children, and is rare in adults or in children under one year of age. The typical phlyctenule appears on the cornea as a pale, grayish-yellow elevation of the epithelium, with a leash of vessels running from the conjunctiva to it. There may be one or many phlyctenules, and they may be at the margin or at or near the center of the cornea. The nearer they are to the center of the cornea the graver the prognosis. Pain in and around the eye, severe photophobia and blepharospasm are marked symptoms, the patient seeking the darkest room and burying his face in any nearby object. In some children it is only with great difficulty that the eye can be examined. In most cases this can only be accomplished by some one taking the child upon his lap and holding its hands, while the surgeon places its head between his knees, taking the precaution to first place a towel across them. Holding the child's head firmly in this position, he should press the upper eyelid gently but firmly upward and backward, with his forefinger near the edge of the lid, the lower lid being pressed backward and downward with the thumb. In most cases the eyeball will roll upward hiding the cornea from view; this difficulty can sometimes be overcome by telling the patient to open the other eye, or by waiting a few moments, when the superior rectus will become fatigued and the eye will roll downward. When the patient is very unruly it is best to give a few whiffs of chloroform; then open the eyelids and turn the cornea into view with a pair

of fixation forceps. The surgeon should not be deterred from making a thorough examination. Hyperaemia and lachrymation are generally present. In some children the eyelids are swollen and the conjunctiva oedematous with a muco-purulent discharge, so that the phlyctenule can be easily overlooked. Phlyctenular keratitis may go through all its stages in from eight to fourteen days. There is great tendency to relapse, phlyctenules reappearing at any time for many months. The pathological changes are an aggregation of cellular elements around terminal nerve fiber. This exudation takes place under the epithelium, and it is the cause of the cone-shaped elevation. As the disease progresses the epithelium over the cone breaks down, leaving an ulcer which may be slow to heal, and may tend to spread superficially or to penetrate deeply, sometimes causing perforation of the cornea; but under treatment phlyctenular ulceration of the cornea generally heals rapidly. If the phlyctenules are superficial, the remaining scar may be of very slight density, and may not interfere with vision or cause any deformity. If they have penetrated deeply the scar will be dense, and if near the center of the cornea it may cause great impairment of vision. If the ulcer perforates the cornea, the iris may become adherent in the cicatrix (see ulcers of the cornea). All these patients should be put on a diet consisting largely of good meat, milk and eggs. They should spend a large part of the time in the open air, and should sleep in large airy rooms which receive plenty of sunlight during the day. Cold salt water baths should be given them three times a week, and the parent or person in charge should be made to understand that they are unhealthy children, notwithstanding they are often large and fat. The exudation within the phlyctenule sometimes breaks down and forms pus before the epithelial covering disintegrates; this form is called pustular keratitis. It runs the same course as the phlyctenular form, and in appearance differs from it only by the elevations being yellow and spherical instead of cone-shaped. The victims of phlyctenular keratitis are generally those who live and sleep in dark, close rooms, and are fed on oatmeal, potatoes, tea and beer, and the children who are nursed long after they should be weaned. The first step in the treatment is to have the child weaned, the eyes kept clean and protected from strong light. This latter can be best accomplished by having the patient wear smoke-colored glasses arranged so as to subdue all the light that enters the eye; this will encourage them to play out of doors. A one five-hundredth solution of Eserine dropped into the eye three times a day will be found of great value in hastening the healing of the ulcers, and in relieving the photophobia by contracting the pupil and reducing the tension of the eyeball. As iritis is seldom a complication in this disease it is generally safe to use Eserine. The remedies most frequently indicated are Puls, ix when there is marked photophobia, with great desire to rub the eyes. Stinging, tearing pains in the eye. Lids swollen, with burning and itching. Thick discharge, which does not excoriate the lids or face. Calc. phos. ix. The cases in which this remedy has given the best results are those in which the patient is more or less indifferent to diffuse daylight, but very sensitive to direct sunlight or artificial light. They are generally large, white, fat children. A hard swollen upper lip without any perceptible local cause is a good indication for this remedy. It is to be given three times a day, and continued for a long time. Merc. dulc. 6x. Indolent forms in which the tissue changes are very slow, especially when the wings of the nose are swollen and sore and the breath very foul. Merc. corr. 6x. When the inflammatory symptoms are marked; the eyeballs hot and dry; the conjunctiva very red, and the ulcer showing a tendency to penetrate the cornea; the patient, seeming to suffer great agony, is very restless and sensitive to bright light. Hepar sulph. 3x. The patients for whom this remedy is indicated are sensitive to touch; the discharge is purulent; the lids swollen and excoriated. The phlyctenules assume the pustular form, and the ulcerations spread superficially and may involve a large part of the cornea. Sulphur 3x will be found to be a most excellent remedy when the patient complains of sticks in his eyes, especially if he has suffered from previous attacks of the disease. Remember that this disease is very apt to return even after the patient seems to be perfectly well.

Abscess of the Cornea.

Synonyms: Circumscribed suppuration of the cornea; Suppurative keratitis.
Abscess of the cornea is most frequently found in those persons whose occupation exposes them to infective injuries of the cornea. Injuries made by the finger nail, or by stacks of grain or hay bruising the cornea, are frequently followed by abscess. It sometimes occurs in debilitated subjects without any known external injury or infection. It may occur from severe conjunctival affections and also during the course of smallpox. A typical abscess of the cornea is generally located in the center of this membrane; it appears like a yellowish-gray disk, thinner at the center than at the circumference, the most opaque part being in the direction in which the ulcer is spreading. The pus is situated in the deep layer of the cornea. It is differentiated from ulceration of the cornea by the fact that the epithelium covering it is intact, and from non-suppurative keratitis by its yellow color and by the surface of the cornea being either elevated or depressed, depending upon the stage of the abscess. The symptoms are those common to nearly all forms of keratitis, such as injection of the peri-corneal zone, hyperaemia of the conjunctiva, pain, photophobia and lachrymation. In addition to these symptoms pus is, as a rule, found in the anterior chamber, and its presence constitutes hypopion. A cloudiness of the cornea may be present, and iritis is almost certain to appear at an early stage if the suppuration is at all severe. The pus in the anterior chamber comes from the cornea or iris, or both. Abscesses of the cornea may be very small and superficial and be limited to its superficial layer, or they may involve the whole of the membrane, and may even extend to the inner tunics of the eye and result in a general panophthalmitis. They general-

ly break on the anterior surface of the cornea, forming an ulcer from which the dead material may be thrown off and healing result by the formation of a more or less dense cicatrix, or the ulceration may extend deeply and perforate the cornea, and if the eye is not lost it may heal by the iris becoming adherent in the cicatrix; this condition is termed leucoma adherens. The pathological changes in abscess of the cornea are the same as in abscess of other parts of the body. This trouble must always be treated as a grave malady, as it nearly always leaves the sight impaired.

Treatment: Put the patient to bed, bandage the eye, keep it clean with a wash of one-tenth thousandth solution of Merc. corr. If iritis is present keep the pupil dilated. Scopolamine is probably the best mydriatic in these cases, as it seems to have the power of reducing the tension of the eyeball. One drop of a one-half per cent, solution may be dropped into the eye every two hours if the trouble is severe. Hepar sulph. 3x is the only remedy I have found of value; give it three times a day. For abscesses that spread in spite of this treatment — and they are very rare — the galvano-cautery may have to be used or an iridectomy made.

Ulcers of the Cornea.

Ulcers of the cornea vary from the simple traumatic ulcers, that show no tendency to spread and that heal in a few days, to the malignant ulcerations that tend to the destruction of the entire cornea and often result in total loss of sight, shrinkage of the eyeball, and even endanger the other eye by sympathetic inflammation. Ulceration of the cornea appears under a great variety of forms, designated by the following terms: Phlyctenular ulcers, Fascicular ulcers, Catarrhal ulcers, Trachomatous ulcers, Central non-irritating ulcers, Ulcers due to purulent and diphtheritic conjunctivitis, Traumatic ulcers, Serpiginous ulcers, Rodent ulcers, Hypopion keratitis, Ring ulcers, Annular ulcers, Facet ulcers, Recurrent vascular ulcers, Crescentic ulcers, Danderitic ulcers, Indolent ulcers, Sloughing ulcers, Clear ulcers, Asthenic ulcers, Creeping ulcers, etc., etc.

All of these forms may be divided into three classes:

Those that tend to destruction.

Those that tend to healing.

Those remaining stationary.

The destructive forms may be vascular or non-vascular. They may spread superficially, or they may extend deeply and perforate the cornea. They may involve the whole cornea, or any part of it, and may extend in a most irregular manner. They may destroy the cornea or the eye, (1) by death of the superficial layers; (2) by perforation of the cornea, resulting in adhesion of the iris, the formation of staphyloma or fistula of the cornea; (3) by destructive changes set up in the iris or lens; (4) by the ulceration extending around the margin of the cornea, cutting off its nutrition and so causing it to die *en masse* or to shrink and become flattened. These destructive forms of ulceration generally occur in debilitated subjects and are in all probability infective in character.

Progressive Ulcers.

These may be recognized by the grayish-yellow color of their bases and edges, by the grayish zone of infiltration which surrounds them, and generally by the inflammatory symptoms that accompany them. The asthenic ulcer, though a very dangerous form, is not accompanied by inflammatory symptoms. When the ulcer tends to heal the grayish deposits disappear, and the surface and edges of the ulceration become transparent. Blood-vessels are often seen extending from the limbus toward the ulcer. As healing progresses the ulcer becomes filled with cicatricial tissue, which is of a more or less pearly-white color, depending upon the depth of the ulceration; the deeper the ulcer the more dense will be the scar. The scar tissue finally becomes covered with epithelium. If the ulcer has perforated the cornea, and the iris heals in the wound, the scar may be more or less pigmented.

Treatment: If iritis is not present the pupil should be kept contracted by a one-fifth per cent, solution of Eserine, one drop to be put into the eye four times a day. The eye should be kept clean by a one two-thousandth solution of Merc. corr. dropped into the eye every hour. Give Hepar sulph. 2x, a grain every two hours, if there is suppuration with great tenderness and swelling of the eyelids. Calc. hypophos. 1x, a grain every hour, in case of asthenic ulcers. A bandage should be applied and the patient kept in bed and fed on the most nourishing diet. In desperate cases, where the ulceration is spreading with great rapidity, the surface and edges may be touched lightly with the galvano-cautery at red heat. This will often arrest the destructive process, but should be done with care and only in extreme cases, Cocaine being used as anaesthetic. If the ulceration is spreading rapidly and the cornea bulging, Saemisch's operation may be resorted to. Kali bich. 3x, a tablet three times a day, is a very valuable remedy in indolent ulceration of the cornea. Brushing such an ulcer with a one one-thousandth solution of Merc. corr. will often convert it into an active ulcer and so lead to repair.

The following remedies have been found of most value in cases of ulceration of the cornea: Hepar sulph. 3x, ulceration with a purulent base and with suppuration around the edges, with hypopion and great tendency to rapid destruction of the corneal tissue. It should be given every hour until the destructive changes are arrested, and then three times a day until healing is completed. Rhus tox. 3x, ulceration of the cornea with marked inflammatory symptoms and oedema of the conjunctiva, with sore, aching pain around the eyes. It should be given every two hours. Kali bich. 3x, in the slow, indolent forms of ulceration, without vascularity of the cornea or injection^ of the conjunctiva, especially if the base and edges of the ulcer seem transparent. It should be given morning and night and continued until the ulceration heals.

Thuja θ, where the loss of tissue is very slight, but the infiltration of the surrounding parts of the cornea is relatively very great. Often the ulcerated spot will be less than a fourth of a millimetre in diameter and the zone of grayish infiltration will exceed five millimetres. A deep, violent injection of portions of the peri-corneal zone will be a further indication. Aurum mur. 3x, when trachoma is a complication; to be given three times a day. For other remedies see various forms of Conjunctivitis and Phylyctenular and Vascular keratitis.

Vesicular Keratitis— Herpes of The Cornea

Keratitis Punctata Superficialis — Filamentous Keratitis — Keratitis Bulbosa.

Herpes corneas occurring during febrile diseases appear as small superficial vesicles; they are transparent and may be found arranged in various forms. Pain, photophobia and lachrymation are marked symptoms, which grow less as the vesicles break. The ulcer that is formed by the rupture of the vesicle is generally shallow and heals under proper care, though neglected cases may become chronic and spread over the cornea. Arsenicum 3x, a tablet three times a day, a bandage to protect the eye and a mydriatic to keep the pupil dilated are the best means of curing this trouble. Herpes zoster cornese occurs when the fifth nerve is implicated. The herpes in this form resemble those of the febrile form, with the exception that the symptoms of irritation do not subside when the vesicles rupture and the ulceration is deeper, runs a more chronic course, is apt to leave dense permanent scars and may lead to loss of sight. The treatment should be the same as simple herpes, but the prognosis should be more guarded.

Keratitis superficialis punctata is characterized by numerous minute punctata spots appearing on the cornea during the course of what seems to be an acute conjunctivitis, either on the first day or at any time within several weeks. It occurs most frequently in children. The symptoms of this trouble resemble those of herpes, but vesicles do not form and ulceration of the cornea seldom takes place. If the punctata occur at the center of the cornea they are apt to affect the sight by reason of grayish spots left by them, which disappear very gradually. Calc. phos. 1x, three times a day, should be given. Vesicular keratitis sometimes occurs without known cause, and recurs periodically.

Filamentous keratitis is a form of the vesicular variety in which, after rupture of the vesicle, small, twisted filaments of fiber are found attached to the ulcerated surface. The treatment is the same as for the herpetic form. Keratitis bulbosa is a form that occurs in eyes that have been destroyed by glaucoma or irido-cyclitis, or where dense maculae cover the cornea. Large blisters or bullae are found on the cornea, accompanied by violent symptoms of irritation. They last for several days and tend to recur with great frequency, the symptoms being very severe with each recurrence. Sometimes cauterization of the surface with Argent, nit. will prevent a recurrence. In other cases, where the eye is useless for vision, it is often best to remove it. Treatment is of very little avail.

Cataract operations, the contact of corrosive liquids or burns of the cornea may cause the formation of vesicles. Apis is the best remedy. The eye should be kept clean and protected from the light, but not bandaged.

Superficial Vascular Keratitis.

Superficial vascular keratitis, including phlyctenular, traumatic and trachomatous pannus, is a type of keratitis that shows no tendency towards suppuration. The inflammatory changes are situated in the epithelial and Bowman's layer. Pannus tenuis, pannus crassus, pannus sarcomatous are terms that are applied to superficial vascular keratitis, the term indicating the amount of inflammatory changes that have taken place; pannus tenuis indicates a case where the change is slight; pannus crassus where the change is marked, and pannus sarcomatous where the cornea resembles a mass of raw flesh.

Phlyctenular pannus occurs in severe attacks of phlyctenular keratitis, when the phlyctenules become confluent and the cornea becomes covered with a more or less vascular membrane. The vessels springing from the superficial vascular zone seem to be continuous with those of the conjunctiva. The treatment is that of phlyctenular keratitis. The pannns disappears rapidly when the primary trouble is cured.

Trachomatous pannus is often a direct extension of granular conjunctivitis, and in that case it is really a trachoma of the cornea. In other cases the pannus seems to have a traumatic origin, the roughened surface of the lids being the exciting cause. This form occurs first in the upper part of the cornea. Most cases of trachomatous keratitis are probably due to both of these causes. The treatment is that of trachoma. Traumatic pannus may be due to any constant friction, incurved eye-lashes being the most frequent cause. This variety is characterized by marked hypertrophy of the corneal epithelium. All forms of pannus tend to disappear when the cause is removed. The prognosis as to the restoration of sight will depend upon the length of time the pannus has lasted and upon the amount of tissue change that has taken place in the cornea. The more recent the disease the more favorable the prognosis. Cases of long standing, even though they appear slight, seldom leave a clear or perfectly curved cornea. Pannus being a secondary disease, the treatment should be directed towards the cause.

Parenchymatous Keratitis.

Interstitial keratitis, Deep keratitis, Diffuse keratitis, Syphilitic keratitis, Uvitis anterior, Secondary keratitis, Deep infiltration of the Cornea and Non-suppurative keratitis are some of the names applied to this disease, which is clinically a well-marked type and runs a characteristic course, though the ultimate pathological changes that constitute it have not been well studied, owing to lack of material. For while the disease is quite common, the eye is seldom destroyed and the patient rarely dies during the course of the disease. It generally attacks both eyes in succession, though

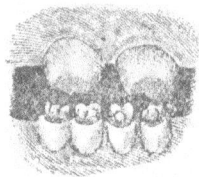

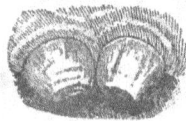

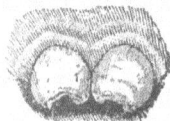

Varieties of Hutchinson's Teeth

often at an interval of months or years. Parenchymatous keratitis occurs most frequently between the ages of five and twenty, though it is sometimes found late in life. The author has seen several cases in negroes between thirty and sixty years of age, and his observation has led him to believe that negroes are more subject to it than white persons. It is nearly always a constitutional disease. The great majority of the sufferers are victims of inherited syphilis. A peculiar formation of the second teeth, more especially of the central incisors, frequently accompanies this condition. The cutting edges of the teeth break down so as to form arches, the convexities of which are directed towards the roots of the teeth. These teeth are called Hutchison's teeth, after the distinguished Jonathan Hutchinson, who first described them. Taken in connection with interstitial keratitis they are considered characteristic of inherited syphilis, though in some cases a history of such inheritance cannot be made out. This disease, or one closely resembling it, has been found in persons suffering from secondary syphilis, but it is doubtful if the specific trouble was a cause of the keratitis, as diseases of the cornea are very rarely caused by primary syphilis. Girls seem to suffer from this disease more frequently than do boys. The symptoms are a haziness of the cornea, which may be diffuse or circumscribed, assuming various forms, sometimes disc-shaped, often like a ring or band, or more frequently very irregular in shape. The color varies from a pale gray to a dense orange, depending upon the amount of exudation and vascularity of the part. An examination by oblique illumination will show this opacity to be situated in the deep portion of the cornea, the superficial layer being almost transparent, though the most superficial part of the epithelium appears to be roughened so that the affected part reflects light irregularly and the cornea has the appearance of a piece of glass upon which moisture has condensed. In the early stages there is no vascularity of the cornea, and some cases run their course without the development of perceptible vessels. In the vascular form the vessels originate from the deep scleral zone and run in the deep parts of the cornea, giving off numerous branches as they proceed towards its center, which they do not quite reach. The center appears like a depressed, grayish spot, which may be mistaken for an ulcer if the presence of the epithelial layer is not recognized.

Sometimes the vessels are so fine and closely meshed and so obscured by the exudation that the affected part looks like an orange-red patch. Pain, photophobia, lachrymation, blepharospasm, hyperaemia of the corneal zone or conjunctivitis may or may not be present. Diminution of the vision is always present, varying from a slight defect to inability to count fingers at a distance of one foot. This failure of vision may be the only symptom that brings the patient to the doctor.

Dilatation of the pupil by the use of a mydriatic will often disclose adhesions of the iris to the lens capsule, and, if the cornea is sufficiently clear, inflammatory changes may be recognized in the anterior part of the choroid; these are often found in the second eye even before the development of the haziness of the cornea. The disease shows no tendency towards suppuration or ulceration. In rare cases, where it has existed for a long time and has been of a very severe character, the cornea may become flattened or staphylomatous. At first the intra-ocular tension is increased; later it is decreased. Without treatment the disease runs an exceedingly chronic course, extending from three months to several years. In the majority of cases the cornea regains its transparency and vision becomes nearly normal, although even when the results are as good as this small dots of opacity may be detected in the cornea when examined by oblique light. The pathological changes in this form of keratitis are infiltration of the deep layers of the cornea by lymphoid elements and serum. The presence of this inflammatory material distends the corneal canals, and the difference between its refractive index and that of the normal tissues of the true cornea is what causes the opacity of the deep portions of the cornea. The roughing of the epithelium is probably due to oedema. In the vascular form there is added to these changes a development of new vessels in the deep cornea; there is sclerosis of the corneal fibers or even the development of new fibrous tissue. Suppuration is not apt to take place. The changes that are found in the choroid and iris are those of disseminated choroditis and plastic iritis.

Treatment: The patient must be placed in the most hygienic surroundings and given the most nourishing food. Atropine sulphate, 1% solution, should be instilled into the eye from time to time to keep the pupil dilated and to prevent adhesions of the iris which may be very easily overlooked on account of the haziness of the cornea. As a rule, iritis is rare in children, except in connection with this form of keratitis. Sometimes the iris will not dilate though there is no iritis present, the condition of the cornea preventing absorption; then the mydriatic must be used persistently, even every two hours until the pupil does dilate. I have tried a great many medicines, and the only one found of any value in shortening the course and preventing the development of this disease in the other eye is Aurum mur. 3x, a grain four times a day, continued until the disease disappears. In some cases the cornea has cleared in two weeks, while in other very severe cases the clearing up process has taken two months. Smoke-colored glasses should be worn when light is painful, and the patient should be kept out of doors as much as possible.

The patient may be told that though the disease is a. chronic one the prospect of restoration of sight is very good. Arlt describes a form of keratitis, parenchymatosa circumscripta, found in rheumatic subjects. It has also been found in patients suffering from chronic malarial poisoning and from traumatism.

Sclerosing Keratitis.

This form is generally found in connection with scleritis, though cases have been described -in which neither scleritis or iritis had at any time existed. Keratitis limited to Descemet's membrane will be described under iritis. (See Diseases of the Iris for treatment of these rare forms of keratitis.)

Keratomalacia.

This is a very rare disease in this country, occurring occasionally in very sick children. The first symptom is night blindness; then the cornea appears very dry, though it may be covered with tears which do not adhere to it, owing to fatty degeneration of the corneal epithelium. Necrosis is very apt to occur, and both eyes are usually implicated. In some cases a certain amount of sight is regained, but generally the eyes are lost and the patient dies. The treatment must depend upon the patient's general condition. The eyes must be kept clean and protected from all irritation.

Keratitis Neuro-paralytica.

This form is a result of paralysis of the trigeminal nerve. It runs a slow course and may assume the form of a purulent keratitis, with subsequent ulceration of the cornea. The prognosis is unfavorable. The treatment is to protect the cornea and restore the function of the nerve. Keratitis resulting from lagophthalmus may start as a simple dryness of the cornea, and result in ulceration and destruction of the cornea and even in panophthalmitis. The treatment is cleanliness and restoration of the function of the eyelids. Until this can be accomplished the eye may be bandaged.

Opacities of the Cornea.

Scars or opacities of the cornea, known as nebula, macula, leucoma and leucoma adherens, are generally the result of ulceration or inflammation. If the opacity is very faint, diffuse and cloud-like, it is termed a nebula. If it is more defined, but translucent, it is termed a macula. If dense and opaque, the term applied is leucoma. If adhesion of the iris has taken place, the term used to indicate the condition is leucoma adherens. Facets of the cornea are old ulcerations that have been incompletely filled with scar tissues. They appear as bright transparent spots that do not correspond with the general curve of the cornea. The impairment of vision due to cicatricial opacities is dependent upon their situation and upon the density of the scar. A large central leucoma may prevent any light from entering the eye, and so cause total blindness. If not so large, or situated to one side of the pupil, it may diminish the amount of light entering the eye and cut off only a part of the field of vision. Nearly every scar of the cornea causes more or less alteration of its curvature, resulting in irregular astigmatism, which may greatly impair sight.

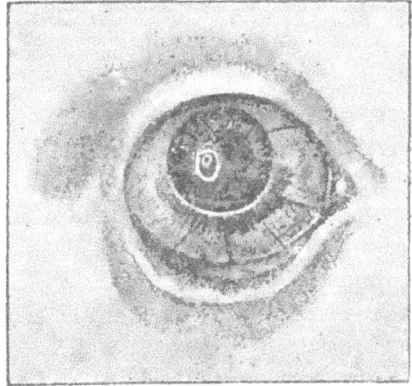

Leucoma Adherens.

Treatment: For leucoma and leucoma adherens, occupying the pupillary space, an iridectomy may be made so as to form a new pupil opposite a clear portion of the cornea. (See Iridectomy, Chapter on Operations.) Macula or nebula, if recent, may be rendered more transparent by the use of Soda bicarb., 10 grains to an ounce of distilled water, a drop to be put into the eye every morning and night. This treatment was used for many years by the late Prof. Liebold. It was from Prof. Liebold that the author learned of its value, and he has used it for many years in several hundred cases, with most gratifying results. The vision and appearance of the eye may often be improved by tattooing the opacity as suggested by de Wecker. (See Operation.) Transplantation of the cornea has been tried in cases where the opacity was of such a size as to make an iridectomy of no value; the results have so far not been satisfactory. Deposits of lime, lead, powder, etc., may sometimes be scraped from the cornea with very good results, after which Aconite 1x, a tablet every hour, should be given, the eye carefully cleaned and then bandaged. Congenital opacities of the cornea are sometimes due to arrest of development, and sometimes to intra-uterine keratitis. They often clear up in a most surprising manner. Zonular opacity of the cornea is due to a degeneration of a band-like portion of the cornea, corresponding to the palpebral opening. It is found in old and feeble persons. The only symptom complained of is loss of sight. Phosphorus, Arsenicum, and Nux vom. are the remedies that will be found to be most useful. They must be given on the general indications, as the eye furnishes no symptoms that guide in prescribing for this condition. Ulcerative, or colloid, fatty or calcareous degeneration may take place in old leucoma. It is termed cicatricial keratitis or atheromatous ulceration.

Treatment: 1:500 solution of Eserine, a drop in the eye morning and night. Bandage the eye and give Hepar sulph. 3x, a tablet morning and night. Glaucomatous opacity of the cornea is due to intra-ocular tension. The cornea presents a diffuse cloudy opacity, most dense in the center, which is evidently due to oedema of the epithelial layer. It disappears very rapidly when the tension is relieved.

Ectasia of the Cornea.

Staphyloma, keratectasis, keratoconus and keratoglobus are terms that are applied to protrusion of the cornea. The first two named are due to the giving away of cicatricial tissue, the bulging portion being more or less opaque. The cause of staphyloma is generally some form of corneal trouble that results in perforation of the cornea, the incarceration of the iris in the wound with subsequent cicatrization and protrusion. It may be partial or complete. For treatment see Ulceration of the Cornea. When the cornea alone is involved it is termed keratectasis. This is quite rare, and generally results from an ulceration that has destroyed the outer layer, leaving intact Descemet's membrane, which protrudes, owing to intra-ocular pressure, in which case it is called keratocele. Subsequently scar tissue forms, but not of sufficient strength to resist the intra-ocular pressure. The instillation of a solution of Eserine, a pressure bandage, or slitting the protrusion may be tried if the trouble is progressing. Calc. phos. 1x may be given. Pannus and parenchymatous keratitis are sometimes the cause of keratectasis. Keratoconus is a form of degeneration of the central portion of the cornea which allows it to yield to the intra-ocular pressure, thus changing its curvature to a conical form. When of slight degree this change is more easily recognized by viewing it from the side. Very slight changes can be determined by the reflected image of external objects, being smaller than those of a normal cornea. It is more common in women than in men, and is most frequent between the ages of twelve and twenty, though cases have been found as early as the eighth and as late as the thirty-eighth year. The protrusion progresses to a certain stage; then, as a rule, stops. Ulceration or rupture are not apt to take place, though in the course of time small opacities are found in the more central portions. Near-sightedness and multiple images are the symptoms complained of by the patient. Upon examination a large amount of astigmatism is generally found in addition to the myopia. Lenses to correct the myopia seldom give much help. A stenopaic hole is of value for near vision, but is of very little use for distinct sight when the patient is moving about on account of its limiting the field of vision to a small central area. We know of no treatment that will restore the cornea to its normal curvature. Various operations have been tried, but with little success. If the patient is seen while the disease is in the progressive stage, the condition of his general system should be carefully inquired into and the indicated remedy given. Keratoglobus is a condition where the cornea becomes enlarged in all its diameters. It is one of the conditions of hydrophthalmus. Phthisis corneae is a flattening of the cornea, the result of various diseases of the cornea and uveal tract. Tumors of the cornea are exceedingly rare. They generally extend from the limbus, and attack first the superficial layer, then the deeper ones. The most common forms are sarcoma and epithelioma. Treatment: Removal at once.

Chapter Four - Diseases of The Sclera

Episcleritis.

Synonyms: Scleritis; Simple Scleritis; Superficial Scleritis.

Episcleritis, or superficial scleritis, is a disease that is quite uncommon and generally occurs in elderly people, and in women more than men. It runs a slow course, with great tendency to relapse. The first symptom noticed is a reddish spot appearing on the eyeball, in the space bounded by the insertion of the recti muscles and the margin of the cornea. Later this spot changes to a rounded prominence, the size and elevation of which may vary greatly. The color of this elevated spot is of a violet or purple hue, and it is generally covered by a fine network of vessels. That it is located beneath the conjunctiva and not in it can be proved by moving that membrane over it. The only thing it is liable to be mistaken for is a large phlyctenule. But a phlyctenule is never covered by a network of vessels; it is always of a different color, and, being situated within the conjunctiva, that membrane can not be moved over it. The phlyctenule is more often found at or near the limbus, while the exudation of scleritis is more often found one or two millimeters from it. Hyperaemia of the conjunctiva and injection of the corneal zone may accompany scleritis. The patient may suffer excruciating pain, or the suffering may be so slight that the patient seeks aid simply because his eye looks red. Sometimes the spot is tender, and presents a doughy feel when pressed with a blunt probe. In the course of a few weeks the exudation becomes absorbed, leaving a spot which becomes a slate-gray color, and may slowly fade away. There is no tendency towards ulceration or thinning of the sclera, and bulging does not occur. The annoying feature of this disease is the tendency towards the formation of new spots of exudation even before the first one has disappeared; several may form in this way, until there is a ring of slate-colored spots around the limbus. Both eyes may be affected. Very few microscopical examinations have been made of the eye during the acute stage of episcleritis, so that we do not feel warranted in giving the pathology of the disease. An acute form of diffuse scleritis is recognized by some authors, in which the surface of the sclera is hyperaemic and the eyes water and ache severely. The diagnosis is made by eliminating all symptoms of disease of the iris, ciliary body, cornea and conjunctiva. Some cases of scleritis have been observed where there was only a spot of violet congestion with no sign of exudation, a slate-colored spot appearing after the congestion had subsided. A haziness of the cornea may appear opposite the lesion in the sclera, which disappears with the scleritis. The cause of scleritis is not known, but it occurs in those patients who have suffered for a long time with rheumatism. The cardinal fact to be remembered in the treatment of scleritis is to avoid the use of irritants. If the case is a very severe one the patient should remain in the house, with the eye bandaged. If the case is not so severe, smoke-colored glasses should be worn to protect the eye from dust and strong light. The remedies found most valuable in this disease are,

Thuja θ, a tablet four times a day. Indications: congestion of the white of the eye; stinging pains with injection of the cornea; dim sight; soreness of the eye, remaining a long time after the eye has been touched; lachrymation. Often when the eye does not furnish characteristic symptoms they may be derived from the general system. In the absence of indications for other drugs, give Thuja.

Rhus tox. 3x, three times a day, for soreness around the eye, sharp pain running into the head, aching from exerting the eyes, swollen feeling in the eye, pain in the eyeball on turning the eye and on pressure, itching in the eyeball.

Kali iod. 1x, four times a day; a peculiar pain in a direct line from the external border of one orbit to that of the other; eyeball feels as if in a rubber covering which keeps up a constant contraction. These three remedies have served me well; but each patient should be carefully studied, as symptoms located in some remote part of the body may give a clue to the indicated remedy.

Deep Scleritis.

Synonyms: Sclero-cyclo-iritis; Sclero-keratitis; Sclerotico-chorioiditis anterior; Kerato-scleritis; Uveo-scleritis.

These are some of the terms that have been applied to a form of scleritis that may result in, or be the result of, inflammatory changes in the uveal tract or cornea. It is a far more dangerous and destructive disease than simple scleritis. It is found more frequently among young persons; it is generally limited to one eye and runs a chronic course. The early symptoms may be those of simple scleritis, though the inflammatory changes are apt to be diffuse rather than circumscribed. To these symptoms may be added those of a deep keratitis which affects the margin more than the center of the cornea, and which shows a tendency to result in a permanent sclerosis of that part of the membrane most severely affected. If the keratitis becomes manifest before the scleritis, then the latter disease is considered secondary to that of the cornea and the trouble is termed kerato-scleritis. The same is true of complications of scleritis with diseases of the uveal tract. Cycloscleritis is the most serious type of scleritis; the part of the sclera affected loses its power of resistance to the normal intra-ocular pressure, and, as a result of this weakening, the part protrudes, forming a condition called staphyloma. As a result of the changes, the tension of the eye is very apt to be increased and so lead to further bulging. The eye-sight may be lost in this way, or as a result of iritis or cyclitis. Dislocation or opacity of the lens, fluidity of the vitreous, occlusion or exclusion of the pupil are some of the ways in which cyclitis or iritis destroy vision. The pathological changes in complicated scleritis may include those of deep keratitis, iritis or cyclitis, depending upon which structures are implicated. (See chapters on Iritis and Scleritis.) In treatment, it is essential that the patient should understand that the disease is a very grave one. He should be put to bed, the eyes kept bandaged and the pupil dilated by a mydriatic to prevent adhesions of the iris. Astringents or irritating applications are positively contraindicated. To the remedies mentioned for simple scleritis may be added.

Hepar sulph. 3x, pain in the eyeballs, bruised feeling w r hen touched. Smarting in the external canthus.

Merc. corr. 6x, pain behind the eyeballs, as if they would be forced out. Burning pains in the inflamed part of the sclera.

Aurum mur. 3x, pressure in the eye in the open air, with tearing pain and dread of light; burning, pricking and itching in the eyes; eyelids red and swollen.

Gumma of the Sclera

Gummata of the sclera have been described appearing as small grayish-purple growths in the sclera, with a tendency to recur. The treatment would be that of the tertiary stage of syphilis.

Injuries of the Sclera.

Injuries of the sclera are always grave, no matter in what portion they occur; but injuries that implicate the ciliary body are to be dreaded most on account of the danger of destructive inflammation being set up in the other eye. (See Sympathetic Ophthalmia.) The sclera may be ruptured by a severe blow with a blunt body, and, as a rule, the rupture will take place opposite the point of impact. Such ruptures have generally been found between the corneal border and the equator of the eye. The lens and a portion of the vitreous may escape from the opening and be found under the conjunctiva. In such cases the I lens should not be removed for several days, until the tear in the vitreous has healed, which is determined by the restoration of the normal intra-ocular tension, which is always decreased when an opening exists in the sclera or cornea. In small cuts or punctures of the sclera diminished tension may be the only symptom that will indicate the condition. Cuts of any magnitude should be stitched together by a delicate suture passed through the superficial layers of the sclera. Protruding buds of vitreous will soon become opaque, when they may be snipped off with the scissors. If a large amount of the vitreous has been lost, the eye is almost certain to become atrophic. If the retina has been cut, the contraction of the cicatrix may lead to the detachment of the retina. Panophthalmitis may result from injuries to the sclera. If the injury is at or near the limbus, the iris may protrude. Eserine solution should be instilled into the eye to contract the pupil and drag the iris out of the wound. If the iris should protrude like a bladder, it should be slit with a narrow cataract knife; this will allow the vitreous to escape and so prevent furthur protrusion. After any injury to the sclera the eye should be carefully bandaged, and a small rubber bag filled with ice should be wrapped in a towel and held gently against the eye. Generally for the first twelve hours after the injury Aconite will be indicated. It should be given in the first decimal, every hour, and continued until all_ symptoms of inflammation have passed away. Before the eye is bandaged it should be washed thoroughly with a 1-10,000 solution of Merc. corr.

Ulcers of the sclera are exceedingly rare. The most common tumors are osteoma, fibroma and sarcoma, though as primary lesions these, too, are very rare.

Ectasia and Staphyloma of the Sclera.

Ectasia, or protrusion of the sclera, may include the entire membrane or any part of it. Circumscribed protrusion may be limited to that part between the border of the cornea and the insertion of the recti muscles; this is termed anterior staphyloma. Any part or the whole of the zone may protrude. If the whole or the part of the zone containing the ciliary body is staphylomatous, it is called a ciliary staphyloma. Equatorial staphyloma is confined to the equatorial zone of the eyeball, and in its etiology resembles anterior staphyloma. Both forms are due to a weakening of the sclerotic by inflammatory changes, though traumatism and new growths of the sclera may be the exciting cause, and sometimes the sclera gives way at these places as a result of intra-ocular tension. The sclera is weak at these points owing to its perforation here by the blood-vessels of the interior of the eye. The anterior ciliary arteries enter, and the veins leave, the eye in the ciliary region. The venae vorticosae escape from the eye in the equatorial region. The diagnosis of these forms of staphyloma is easily made by observing the location of the protrusion of the sclera and its color, which is of dark slate, or even bluish-black. In order to diagnose the equatorial form, the eye should be rotated strongly in the direction opposite to the side that protrudes. Intra-ocular tumor, causing protrusion of the sclera, is the only condition likely to be mistaken for any of these forms of staphyloma; but the distinguishing point is the comparative transparency of the true staphyloma, which will admit light when concentrated on its surface. Prognosis as regards cure is bad. If the trouble can be arrested, that is the best that can be hoped for. For this purpose an iridectomy will sometimes answer, but in some cases this operation is rendered impossible by the extensive adhesions of the iris, and that is only one of several complications which may arise. The lens may become dislocated, the retina detached, the eyesight destroyed by secondary glaucoma, which is often caused by, and is the cause of, anterior and equatorial staphyloma. Posterior staphyloma differs from all other forms, and will be described under the head of myopia. A congenital protrusion of the eyeball occurring below the posterior pole of the eye has been described by Ammon under the name of posterior scleral protuberance. It is simply an anomaly and leads to no destructive changes. Total ectasia of the sclera is a disease limited to youth, the entire sclera giving way to intra-ocular tension, which may or may not be greater than normal. It is a very rare disease. An iridectomy may hold it in check. It may follow anterior staphyloma, the eyeball becoming greatly enlarged, protruding even beyond the eyelids, in which case the eyeball should be removed. Pigmentation of the sclera occurs in Addison's disease and also as a congenital anomaly.

Chapter Five - Diseases of the Iris and Ciliary Body

Diseases of those parts of the uveal tract anterior to the ora serrata, consisting of the ciliary body and iris, demand careful study on account of their great importance, their prompt response to treatment, and the sad results that are almost certain to follow a mistaken diagnosis and consequent improper treatment. Inflammation of the iris and ciliary body can not be left to nature to effect a cure, as such a course results at best in a maimed eye. Though the iris and ciliary body are so intimately connected anatomically that it is doubtful if one portion of the anterior part of the uveal tract can be inflamed without, to some extent, affecting the entire structure, yet, clinically, it is of importance to distinguish between inflammations apparently limited to the iris and inflammations implicating the ciliary body, termed respectfully iritis and cyclitis.

Cyclitis is a far more serious disease than iritis on account of the functional importance of the ciliary body. Iritis is more common than cyclitis. When both the iris and ciliary body participate in the inflammation, the disease is termed irido-cyclitis. Iritis is a very common disease in adult life, and very rare in children under ten years of age, except as a complication of parenchymatous keratitis or as a result of injury. It is frequently found in young girls at puberty, and it is seldom found after the age of seventy. Iritis has been studied under a great variety of terms by various writers. Among the most common of these terms are: Arthritic, Diabetic Gelatinous, Gonorrhoeal, Gouty, Gummatous, Parenchymatous, Plastic, Primary, Recurrent, Relapsing, Rheumatic, Scrofulous, Serous, Simple, Spongy, Suppurative, Syphilitic, Specific, Traumatic, Tubercular, and Variolous Iritis. For the practical physician these various forms can well be included under the terms Plastic, Suppurative and Serous Iritis, and under these three heads we will consider them.

Hyperaemia of the Iris and Plastic Iritis.

Hyperaemia of the iris, in addition to being the first symptom of inflammation, is sometimes found as an independent affection and frequently as a complication of disease of the cornea, sclera, ciliary body or orbital cellular tissue. It is characterized by change of color of the iris, due to the excessive amount of blood in its tissue, causing a blue iris to become greenish and a brown one to become a reddish brown; these changes may be very slight or very marked. The pupil will be contracted and the iris sluggish in its movements, both in response to light and to mydriatics and myotics. To test the pupillary response to light, the eye not under examination should be closed and covered by some opaque substance; then the eye under examination should be rapidly covered and uncovered, and the dilatation and contraction of the pupil noted. If doubt exists as to its movements, the examination should be made by artificial light in a darkened room, the light being concentrated by a convex lens and the eye alternately illuminated by this concentrated light and shaded by the shadow of the lens. This method gives very striking results. In simple hyperaemia the aqueous humor will be clear, and the surface of the iris will present its normal lustre; and when the pupil is dilated by a mydriatic it will present no irregularities. Treatment of hyperaemia of the iris should be that of simple iritis, for we have no way of determining simple hyperaemia from that which is the first stage of iritis. Among the causes of iritis syphilis ranks first, fully 65 per cent, of all cases being due to this cause. Rheumatism, including the gonorrhoea! form, is the next greatest cause. Traumatism is a frequent factor. It may occur during smallpox, diabetes, tuberculosis and other diseases. Sometimes no cause can be discovered. Kerato-iritis is a term applied when the inflammation has extended from the cornea to the iris. The pathological changes that take place in plastic iritis are analogous to inflammations 01 serous membranes in general, modified by the location and function of the iris. The first stage is that of congestion followed by an exudation of plastic inflammatory liquid containing leucocytes and red blood corpuscles, which may be relatively very few, or their number may be so great that the exudate will look like a blood-clot. This plastic exudation shows a great tendency to coagulate, sometimes in the form of a gelatinous mass, which looks like a crystalline lens lying in the lower part of the anterior chamber. This has given rise to the term gelatinous or spongy iritis. In the forms called parenchymatous, gummy or condylomatous, the exudation is composed mostly of cellular elements, appearing as reddish-brown nodules ranging in size from that of a small pin's head to that of a pea. They are similar in structure to gumma found in other parts of the body, and are made up of connective tissue cells and young cicatricial tissue, which become necrosed and undergo caseation, followed by absorption; healing takes place by the formation of cicatricial tissue, a scar occupying the place of the gumma. Gumma are generally situated near the pupillary margin, though sometimes near the periphery of the iris. One or more may exist at the same time. They make their appearance most frequently between the secondary and tertiary stage of syphilis. This is the only form of iritis that we can say positively is due to syphilis. The inflammatory exudation poured out in plastic iritis tends to gravitate to the most dependent portion of the aqueous chamber. In cases of slight or moderate degree of severity the exudation coagulates in the form of small particles. If these particles find lodgment between the posterior surface of the iris and the surface of the anterior capsule, so as to touch both these surfaces, then these surfaces adhere at these points; this union is of no great degree of strength, and may be easily broken. In a short time inflammatory cells from the iris proliferate at this point of union, replacing the lymph by new formed fibrous tissue, which causes the union to become very firm and of a permanent character. Synechia is the term applied to adhesions of the iris to any part of the walls of the aqueous chamber. If the adhesion is between the iris and the anterior capsule of the lens it is called posterior synechia. If the pupillary margin is completely adherent, the condition is called annular or circular synechia. If the entire iris is adherent to the

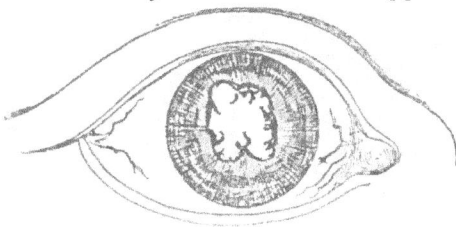

Iritis with Posterior Synechia.

capsule of the lens, it is termed complete synechia. Adhesion between the iris and the posterior surface of the cornea is called anterior synechia. A contracted pupil and a quiescent iris are favorable conditions for the formation of posterior synechia, for the reason that when the pupil is small the iris rests on the anterior capsule of the lens. When the pupil is widely dilated the iris floats free in the aqueous humor, consequently the particles of coagulated fibrin can find no place of lodgment, and soon undergoes disintegration and absorption. The movements of the iris tend to break adhesions before they become firmly adherent, and so the majority of adhesions form during sleep. As a rule, adhesions do not form at the pupillary edge of the iris but at a slight distance from it, at the place of contact between the posterior surface of the iris and the lens capsule. In very severe cases of iritis, especially when complicated by cyclitis, the exudation coagulates in large masses, and sometimes over the entire posterior surface of the iris, resulting in adhesions which may involve the entire iris. Sometimes synechiae form around the pupillary margin in a complete zone; then the aqueous humor accumulates behind the iris, and, being unable to escape on account of the adhesions around the pupillary edge, causes the rest of the iris to bulge forward, giving rise to the condition called crater iris. The formation of a false membrane occupying the pupillary space is due to coagulation of the plastic lymph, forming a laminated structure of fibers containing blood-corpuscles and other cells between its meshes. This membrane is closely adherent to the anterior capsule of the lens. Its attachment to the iris may be complete, or it may be adherent only at several points. If the adhesion of the membrane to the iris is complete, the result will be occlusion of the pupil. Although this membrane is of loose structure, it greatly interferes with vision. The further changes that take place in plastic iritis are atrophy of the true tissue of the iris and its replacement by a low grade of fibrous tissue. This change may be limited to a small part of the iris, or it may involve the entire membrane, or even the whole eye, depending upon the severity of the attack and the method of treatment adopted.

The symptoms of plastic iritis are injection of the pericorneal zone of vessels, which appear as a more or less rosy band surrounding the cornea. The depth of this congestion can be determined by pressure with the ringer through the eyelid; if it is superficial or conjunctival, the blood will be driven out and the part pressed will look pale; but if the congestion is deep, involving the ciliary vessels, pressure will have little effect. In addition to the congestion of the peri-corneal zone there will be marked hyperaemia of the conjunctiva. This last symptom is generally found in severe cases of iritis. There will be a change of color in the iris, a reddish tint being added, causing a blue iris to become greenish and a brown one to become reddish brown. There will be noted a loss of the normal brilliancy of the iris, with haziness of the aqueous humor, due to the inflammatory exudation contained in it. In the spongy forms the exudation may coagulate, forming a mass which resembles a dislocated lens. In the gummatous forms reddish-brown nodules are found projecting from the anterior surface of the iris. The pupil will dilate and contract sluggishly, as explained under Hyperaemia of the Iris. The cardinal symptom of iritis is the presence of synechia, manifested by an irregular shape of the pupil, which is best demonstrated by instilling between the lids a 1:100 solution of Atropine sulphate.

Pain is a symptom which varies greatly in different forms and in different persons. It may be located in the eye or more frequently around the orbit, or both the face and head may be involved; it is generally worse at night. It may be so severe that the patient will lose all control of himself and become frantic. On the other hand, it may be so slight that it scarcely attracts attention, the disease being allowed to run its course without medical care, the eye becoming hopelessly damaged by the formation of synechia. Photophobia and lachrymation may or may not be present. In the very early stages vision may

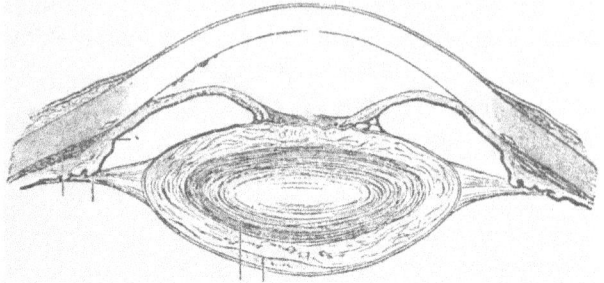

Seclusion and Occlusion of Pupil. Magnified 5x1 (after Fuchs).

not be impaired. When the aqueous becomes turbid the sight becomes hazy. When the pupil becomes occluded the sight may be reduced to a mere perception of light. Swelling of the eyelids is sometimes found in very severe cases, but it nearly always indicates implication of the ciliary body (iridocyclitis). The course of plastic iritis may be acute or chronic, its duration varying from five days to many weeks. In some cases relapses are frequent, more particularly in those in which rheumatism — and especially gonorrhoeal rheumatism — is the etiological factor. Some patients suffering with gonorrhoeal rheumatism will have an attack of iritis with every exacerbation of the rheumatic trouble, which shows itself by an increase of the gleety discharge and an inflammation of the knee-joint. To cure the iritis the gleet must be cured.

In the treatment of plastic iritis medicinal substances are used for two purposes, mechanical and curative. The mechanical treatment is of great importance. Its object is to prevent the iris from adhering to the capsule of the lens, and in case adhesions have already formed to break them and prevent others from forming. This is accomplished by keeping the pupil dilated until the inflammatory symptoms have disappeared. The mydriatic most commonly used is Atropine sulphate, and in most cases it is to be preferred to all others on account of its sustained action, and because it can be readily obtained in a pure state. A drop of a one per cent, solution should be placed on the surface of the conjunctiva of the lower lid near the outer corner of the eye, the lid being drawn gently downward and held in that position for a moment, the patient in the meantime holding his head so that the outer canthus is lower than the inner one. This position will tend to prevent the solution entering the tear passage, and so passing to the throat, and consequently will lessen the liability of enough of the drug being absorbed to produce symptoms of poisoning. These sometimes arise when the solution is used frequently, and in some rare cases where the patient is very susceptible to the drug a single drop may cause unpleasant symptoms. In an acute case of plastic iritis, Atropia should be dropped in the eye every two hours during the active stage, and as the disease subsides it should be used every three, four, six or twelve hours, being guided by the state of the pupil, which should be kept widely dilated until the inflammatory symptoms have disappeared. In cases where the adhesions are so strong that they resist the action of Atropia, a drop of a one per cent, solution of Hydro-bromate of Hyoscine may be dropped in the eye in the same manner indicated for Atropia. Hyoscine hydrobromate is a very powerful drug, and should be used only by the physician himself. The dilatation obtained by Hyoscine should be kept up by Atropia in the manner described above. Neglected cases, where the iritis has existed for several days before being seen by the physician, and where the adhesions are broad and strong, or when the attack is so violent that adhesions form in spite of the mydriatic and resist its power to break them, require the administration of some drug that has the power of destroying the new-formed tissue. For such cases the writer has found Merc. dulc. ix of great value, given in one-grain doses every hour for two or three days. At about the time constitutional symptoms of the drug manifest themselves, the adhesions will generally give way and the pupil will dilate. The Mercurius should then be discontinued, but the Atropia continued, the indicated remedy being substituted for the Mercurius. It must be understood that Merc, dulc. given in this way is not given as a remedy for the constitutional disease, but as a destructive agent for the purpose of destroying the new-formed tissue that causes the adhesion. The evils resulting from extensive synechia are so great that the writer believes this course of treatment justified, even if the patient does suffer some discomfort for a short time. The symptoms produced are those of a severe watery diarrhoea, a putrid odor from the mouth, and in some cases small ulcers will form in the mouth. The symptoms pass away very rapidly when the drug is discontinued. To effect a cure of iritis the mechanical methods must always be supplemented by the homoeopathic remedy, as indicated by the symptoms. Among the remedies of most value in iritis are Merc. corr. 3.x, when the eyes are sparkling and red, with burning and dryness; marked photophobia; pain behind the eyeballs, as if they would be forced out; tearing pain near the root of nose, pain worse at night. To be given every two hours during the acute stage, then three times a day. Hepar sulph. 3x, pain in the eyeball, with a feeling of soreness when the eyeball is touched; swelling of the eyelids; patient very sensitive, will start when the eye is barely touched; no marked aggravation at night; iritis that runs a slowcourse. To be given at first every two hours, later three times a day. Rhus tox. 3x, soreness around the eyes; sharp pains running into the head; requires exertion to move the eyeballs; rheumatic iritis. To be given every hour at first, then three times a day. Thuja θ, biting pain in the eyes; burning pain on upper surface of eyeball; eyeballs tender to touch; a soreness remains for some time after they are touched, even if the finger is immediately removed. This is an excellent remedy in the rheumatic forms of iritis, especially when there is a tendency towards the cornea becoming involved. To be given three times a day until the iritis is cured. Cinnabaris 3x, in simple plastic iritis, when the marked symptom is a pain running from the inner to the outer canthus, seemingly to the bone. To be given every two hours. Cases of iritis are sometimes seen in which this will be the only subjective symptom.

Suppurative Iritis.

Suppurative iritis is rarely found as a primary disease, being more often the result of disease of the cornea or the ciliary body and choroid. In the latter case it forms one of the symptoms of panophthalmitis. Traumatism is probably one of the most frequent causes of suppuration of the iris. It is often met with as one of the results of unsuccessful cataract operation. Simple primary suppurative inflammation is the least grave of all the various forms of iritis. The pathological changes that distinguish this form of iritis from the

plastic variety is a rapid disintegration and death of the exudated inflammatory elements. The tissues of the iris in and around the inflamed area may
also participate in this disintegration, and, as a result, a part or whole of the
iris may become atrophic. If the exudation and disintegration are localized
within the tissue of the iris, the condition is termed abscess of the iris. The
pus which escapes from the inflamed iris finds its way to the bottom of the
anterior chamber. Its presence there gives rise to the condition which is
termed hypopion. Even in the most violent cases of suppurative iritis some of
the plastic exudation will escape death, and may cause synechia. Any of the
symptoms given in plastic iritis may be present in the suppurative form, in
addition to the symptom that gave it its character, viz: pus within the iris,
distinguished by yellowish nodules situated near the pupillary border. These
nodules can be distinguished from those of gummatous iritis by their color,
which is a cream-yellow, the gumma being of a reddish-brown tint. The presence of pus in the anterior chamber is easily made out, and can be distinguished from hypopion due to keratitis by the absence of disease of the cornea.

Treatment: Atropia to dilate the pupil, which is not so difficult to keep dilated as in plastic iritis. A bandage to protect the eye, and rest in bed. Hepar
sulph. 3x three times a day. If the disease is secondary to keratitis or choroiditis, see treatment of those diseases. It is very seldom, if ever, that a homoeopathic physician will have to resort to paracentesis in uncomplicated suppurative iritis.

Serous Iritis.

Synonyms: Serous Cyclitis; Serous iiido-cyclitis; Uvitis serosa; Keratitis
punctata; Descemititis; Aquo capsulitis. This is a disease that is seldom limited to the iris, and in some cases the iris is so slightly involved in the inflammatory changes that no appreciable symptoms are presented by this
membrane. Then the case is termed serous cvclitis, on account of the ciliary
body seeming to be more deeply involved than the other structures of the
eye. The pathological changes are a marked exacerbation of the serous exudation with a limited amount of plastic material, proliferation and disintegration of the epithelial cells of the iris, of Descemet's membrane and of the tissues of the iritic angle. Synechia is not common and forms very slowly. The
pigment cells seem to disintegrate, free pigment being found in the aqueous
humor and in the corneal deposits. These deposits are generally found on the
posterior surface of the cornea, and are often of a pyramidal shape, with base
directed downward; some of them seem to be attached only at the apex,
which allows the base to change its position as the head is moved. They are
made up mainly of disintegrated epithelial cells, with pigment scattered
through the mass. Inflammatory changes have been found in Descemet's
membrane, at its point of union with these bodies. This form was termed
descemititis, but later observations have shown that even in these cases the

corneal symptoms are only a part of the disease, the ciliary body, choroid and retina being involved. A post-mortem examination made by Max Knies in a case of serous iritis showed the entire uveal tract, the sheath of the optic nerve, the retina and optic disk to be in a state of inflammation. The symptoms of serous iritis are those of a low grade of plastic iritis, with the exception that the pupil is not contracted but dilated. There is an increase in depth of the anterior chamber, deposits on the posterior surface of the cornea, an increase or decrease of the intra-ocular tension, depending upon the stage of the disease and the extent to which the ciliary body is involved. Posterior polar cataract may appear at a later stage, and the disease may terminate in atrophy. The condition of the choroid or retina can not be made out unless the aqueous and vitreous are clear; the former is nearly always turbid, and the latter is very apt to become so sooner or later in the course of the disease. Serous iritis is oftenest found in persons suffering from grave disease, more especially in those who are anaemic. It is more common among women than among men, and menstrual troubles have been mentioned as a factor. It runs a slow chronic course. The prognosis should be guarded until the case has been under observation long enough to determine whether it is responding to remedies.

Treatment: Have the patient live out of doors as much as possible, avoiding dampness and severe cold, at the same time avoid keeping him too warmly clothed. Good nourishing food should be given, and smoke-colored glasses prescribed. A mydriatic should be used to prevent the formation of synechia. It will not be necessary to use the mydriatic as energetically as in plastic iritis — use only often enough to keep the pupil dilated. A one-half per cent, solution of Scopolamine will in all probability be the best mydriatic for these cases. Among the remedies found most useful are Gels, 1x, when the patient complains of great heaviness, as after night-watching. Pupils dilated. Sclerotic congested. Pain in the orbit with fulness. Bryonia θ, eyeballs very sensitive to touch. Pain much worse when moving the eyes. Throbbing in the eyeballs.

Functional Disturbances of the Iris.

Mydriasis — a persistent dilatation of the pupil. Myosis — a persistent contraction of the pupil. Hippus — a clonic spasm of the iris, sometimes called Nystagmus of the iris. Iridodonesis — a trembling of the iris. Anisocoria — an inequality in the diameters of the pupils.

Mydriasis may be spastic or paralytic. The spastic form is due to affections of the sympathetic nerve. The paralytic form is due to weakness of the sphincter muscle of the iris, which is supplied by a branch of the third nerve. The causes of mydriasis are many; they may be central or local.

It is sometimes caused by diphtheria, in which case the iris regains its function after a few weeks. Gels. 3x, three times a day, will hasten the cure. Mydriasis due to syphilis is the least favorable, sometimes resisting all treatment. Aurum mur. 3x is the remedy that has given me most satisfaction in such cases. Traumatism, generally in the form of a contusion, is a common cause. Unless the iris has been torn the cases caused by traumatism will recover promptly under Arnica 3x or Aeon. 3x, three times a day. Increased intra-ocular tension is a cause, or, more strictly speaking, mydriasis is a symptom of increased intra-ocular tension. Treatment should be directed to the cause of the increased tension. (See Glaucoma, Tumors, etc.) Mydriasis may result from fright, from irritation of the skin or mucous membrane, and it may be present when the patient is blind. The most common form is the toxic. It may be local, as when a drug is dropped into the eye. Mydriasis from Atropia is generally greater than that due to diseases involving the third nerve only. It is supposed that Atropia used locally not only paralyzes the circular muscles of the iris, but irritates the sympathetic nerve; consequently this condition presents a combination of spastic and paralytic mydriasis. Myosis may also be spastic or paralytic. It is common in old age, in spinal diseases and in poisoning by drugs that have a myotic action, such as Eserine, Pilocarpin, etc. In spinal myosis the pupil, while not reacting to light, will react to accommodation and convergence. Anisocoria is sometimes found where there exists a great difference in the refraction of the two eyes. Myopic eyes generally have large pupils. Hippus is a rare condition, and its cause is not well understood. Iridodonesis is due to the iris losing its support from the lens, which may be absent or dislocated, or it may have lost a part of its support by reason of the vitreous becoming fluid. A slight motion has been observed in the peripheral portion of the iris of eyes that were otherwise normal. Functional affections of the iris, as seen in diseases of the nervous system, are most interesting, and will repay careful study. The author regrets that the size of this book limits the subject to this very brief sketch.

Injuries of the Iris.

Iridodialysis, or separation of the iris from its ciliary attachment, may result from an injury. This rupture is beyond repair; if of slight extent it will cause no inconvenience. If the tear invades the visual area, the eye will have two pupils and consequent monocular diplopia when the eye is not focused true. The relief for this is found in iridectomy, the bridge of tissue being divided so as to throw the two pupils into one. (See chapter on Operations.) The iris may be completely torn from its attachments, and appear as a ball in the anterior chamber, or, if the sclerotic has also been torn, it may escape from the eye. The absence of the iris is termed irideremia. Radiating lacerations and inversion of the iris may be the result of traumatism. In general, injuries to the iris are best treated by bandaging the eye and applying a rubber bag filled with ice, which should be kept applied as long as there is any danger of inflammation, usually from three to seven days. Aeon, 1x, a tablet every hour, should be given. If the injury is near the ciliary attachment, Atropia should be dropped in the eye to dilate the pupil and so relieve the strain.

In radiating lacerations and inversion of the pupil, Eserine should be used to contract the pupil. Foreign bodies in the iris are best removed by an iridectomy, unless they can be easily grasped by the forceps.

Tumors of the Iris.

Tumors of this membrane are very rare. They include tuberculous growths, which may exist as a single tumor or as multiple minute nodules, to which the term miliary tuberculosis is applied. This condition is nearly always secondary to tuberculous trouble in some other part of the body. The tubercles appear as pale, pinkish-gray tumors, and, as a rule, they destroy the eye by their growth. They are found in young people, and the only treatment is removal of the eye. Sarcomata are to be distinguished by their dark color and marked vascularity. If they are small and confined to the iris they may be removed by an iridectomy, taking care to remove sufficient tissue to get out all of the growth. If the growth is large, the eye should be removed. Sometimes simple pigmented growths appear on the iris, and they may be mistaken for sarcoma. The rate of growth may distinguish them from sarcoma, but in cases where doubt exists removal is to be advised; then a diagnosis can readily be established by a microscopic examination. Cysts of the iris are of two kinds — serous and pearl. The contents of the serous cyst are transparent and its walls thin, the whole growth appearing translucent. In the pearl cyst the contents are opaque, looking like tallow. The cause of cyst of the iris is almost always an incised wound of the eye. It is supposed that the penetrating instrument carries epithelial cells from the eyelids or conjunctiva, or even a cilia, and its root may be carried in and deposited in or on the ins. These cells, rapidly proliferating, form a mass within which serous exudation takes place, converting it into a cyst. If not removed it will continue to grow until the eye is destroyed. It may be removed with surrounding portions of the iris, care being taken not to break the cyst's wall, for if any portion is left the tumor will be reproduced. Cysticerci have been found in the anterior chamber. Other growths of the iris are sometimes found, such as lepra nodules, myomata, etc. Their character can be determined only after removal, and then by the aid of a microscope.

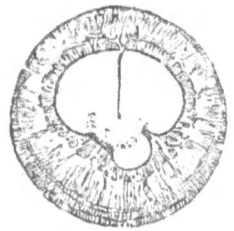

Posterior synchiae of the remains of a pupillary membrane. 2x1

Congenital Anomalies of the Iris.

Aniridia — absence of the iris. Coloboma — an imperfect iris. Persistent pupillary membrane. Corectopia — a displacement of the pupil. Variation of color of the irises.

Coloboma of the iris exists as a triangular-shaped opening, with its apex rounded. It extends from the pupillary edge of the iris towards and even into the ciliary attachment. Coloboma of the choroid is often associated with this, and sometimes the edge of the lens is found notched. Almost always the defect is in the lower edge of the iris. Persistent pupillary membrane appears as a more or less opaque membrane crossing the center of the pupil. It is attached to the anterior surface of the iris by fibrous bands. It sometimes consists of only a few threads of membrane.

Diagram showing the principal nerves and blood vessels of the eyeball. Pathological membranes can be distinguished from this anomaly by the fact that they are attached to the posterior surface of the iris near its pupillary edge, and that dilatation of the pupil is always impaired, which is not the case in persistent pupillary membrane.

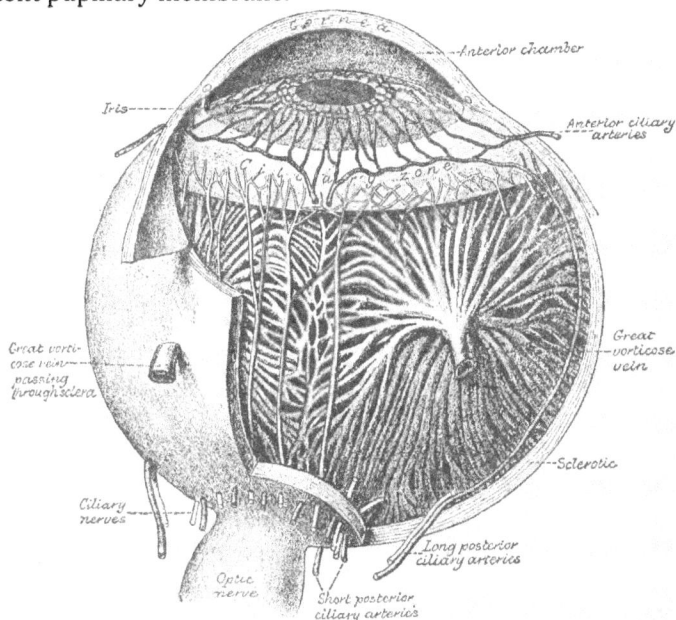

Diagram showing the principal nerves and blood vessels of the eyeball.

Cyclitis.

Inflammation of the ciliary body seldom exists as an independent affection, the iris sooner or later participating in the inflammation. The pathological changes in cyclitis resemble those of inflammation of fibro-muscular structures, such as the heart, and consist of an exudation of fibroplastic material and serum into and from the ciliary body, giving rise to two forms of cyclitis — the serous and the plastic. When the inflammatory cellular exudation undergoes purulent degeneration, we have a third form, called purulent or suppurative cyclitis. On account of the situation and the two-fold function of the ciliary body, cyclitis is a very grave disease. If the plastic exudation that is poured out from its surface invades the vitreous it will coagulate in that structure, forming a mass of fibro-plastic material behind the lens. The subsequent contraction of this mass will cause shrinkage of the anterior part of the vitreous, which in its turn will cause a detachment of the retina, and even of the choroid, with finally shrinkage of the eyeball. Even in cases where the exudation is slight the anterior part of the vitreous may become liquid and the lens may become opaque. The ciliary body supplies the nutrition of these parts. If the plastic exudation should pass into the aqueous chamber behind the iris, that membrane would become adherent to the posterior capsule of the lens, tending to form total posterior synechia and consequent obliteration of the posterior chamber, with all its direful consequences.

Symptoms, Etiology and Course. In addition to the symptoms common to plastic iritis, we find the ciliary region painful to touch; this may vary in amount from slight tenderness to very severe pain. There will be a diminution in the power of accommodation and a haziness of the anterior part of the vitreous. Increased or decreased intraocular tension may appear during the course of the disease, as may also a swelling of the eyelids. The causes of cyclitis are the same as of iritis, with the addition of inflammation of the ciliary region of the other eye; this is a prominent cause, and the inflammation thus set up is called sympathetic inflammation. Cyclitis may run an acute or a chronic course, one or both eyes being affected. It may terminate in recovery with a fair amount of vision, or in complete destruction of the eye. Syphiloma or gumma of the ciliary body may attain great size and cause destruction of the eyeball. Its presence is determined during cyclitis by the appearance of a rapidly growing tumor in the ciliary region. Purulent cyclitis, when not a symptom of panophthalmitis, shows itself by the presence of hypopion without disease of the iris and cornea. Serous cyclitis has been given under the head of serous iritis.

Treatment: The treatment of cyclitis should be same as that of iritis, though even greater care should be exercised. Even in slight cases the patient should be put to bed, his eyes carefully bandaged, and under no condition should he be allowed to use either eye until all symptoms of inflammation have passed away. Keep the pupil dilated, if possible, though when synechia forms, involving, as it generally does in this trouble, the entire posterior surface of the iris, mydriatics seem to be of little value, and persistent use of them may do harm. For gumma of this region large doses of saturated solution of Potassium Iodide should be given in hopes of checking their growth.

Sympathetic Ophthalmitis.

This is a term applied to an inflammation of one eye which has been set up by conditions existing in the other one. In the majority of such cases sympathetic inflammation takes the form of an irido-cyclitis, which may be of the plastic variety. A great many diseases, such as optic neuritis, retinitis, glaucoma, cataract, etc., have also been considered as of sympathetic origin. The lesions that set up sympathetic ophthalmitis are those that involve the ciliary body. Wounds in this region are the most frequent cause, though any injury which primarily or secondarily involves the anterior part of the uveal tract may act as an exciter. An eye destroyed by panophthalmitis is seldom the cause of sympathetic ophthalmitis, though some cases, where calcareous degeneration has taken place, prove exceptions to this rule. The path of transmission and the nature of the exciting cause are disputed points, some authorities believing that irritation of the ciliary nerves is the cause, and others that the optic nerve is the cause and path of the trouble. Still others believe that micro-organisms or septic matter transmitted by the blood-vessels are exciting factors. The theory of transmission of inflammatory material by the lymphatics, as advocated by Max Knies, seems most consistent with clinical observation. However this may be, the fact to be borne in mind is, that the prompt removal of the exciting eye is the best prophylactic. A group of symptoms consisting of sensitiveness of the eye when touched or on movement, pain in and around the eye, weakness of accommodation, photophobia, lachrymation and injection of the circum-corneal zone constitute sympathetic irritation. This may appear at any time, from three weeks to thirty years after the injury to the exciting eye. Sympathetic irritation may be but the early symptom of sympathetic ophthalmitis, or it may constitute the entire malady. In any case, it is promptly relieved, as a rule, by the removal of the offending eye. If uvetis has been established — manifested by symptoms of iridocyclitis, either of the plastic or serous variety — the prospect of relief is not so certain. In every case where an eye has been rendered blind by an injury in the ciliary region, and in all cases where the eyeball is soft, shrunken and painful to touch, enucleation of the eyeball should be made at once. If the patient refuses to submit to the operation, he must be impressed with the importance of placing himself under the observation of a physician as soon as the slightest sign of irritation shows itself, as these eyes may remain quiescent for many years and then suddenly become the cause of sympathetic ophthalmitis. If there is a useful amount of vision in the exciting eye and the second one is already inflamed, removal would not be advisable, as after the disease has run its course the first eye may retain more sight than the second one. Council should be sought before removing the eye. Sympathetic ophthalmitis may run a course so violent that the eye is destroyed within forty-eight hours, or it may run so chronic a course that it presents no marked symptoms of inflammation but only a gradual loss of sight. Some cases are very mild and recover with a fair amount of vision. The prognosis must always be guarded, especially if the exciting eye has not been removed.

Treatment: In addition to what has already been given, the treatment should be the same as for irido-cyclitis. It is very dangerous to make any operation on an eye that has suffered from sympathetic ophthalmitis. Tumors of the ciliary body are very difficult to differentiate, and they generally demand the removal of the eye. Functional troubles of the ciliary body will be considered under the head of Anomalies of Accommodation.

Section Two

Diseases of The Crystalline Lens, Vitreous Body, Choroid, Retina, Optic Nerve. Glaucoma. Anomalies of Refraction, Accommodation and Convergence. Ophthalmoscopy.

Chapter Six - Anatomy and Physiology of the Lens, Vitreous, Choroid, Retina and Optic Nerve

The crystalline lens is a transparent, biconvex body, with rounded edges. Its vertical and horizontal diameters measure about 8 mm., and its antero-posterior diameter about 4 mm. The curve of its anterior surface is that of an ellipsoid, rotated on its short axis. Its radius of curvature varies from 6 to io mm., depending upon the state of accommodation. The curve of the posterior surface is that of a portion of a paraboloid. The change in the radius of curvature of this surface is not great during the act of accommodation, varying from six to about five and a half millimetres. The lens substance belongs to the epithelial group, and consists of long hexagonal fibers, held together by a cement substance. These fibers run in a semi-spherical direction; a fiber starting near the center of one surface, will terminate near the margin of the other surface. As a result of this arrangement, the surfaces of the lens are marked out into sectors by radiating lines. In the young lens there are three well-marked lines on each surface. On the posterior surface one of these lines is directed upward, the other two forming equal angles with it, thus producing a stellate figure with six rays. In the adult lens, other shorter irregular rays may be seen between these. In the early stages of cataract the rays often become well-marked, appearing as black or gray lines, the color depending upon whether they are seen by transmitted or by reflected light. In early life all these fibers contain nuclei; later these nuclei are found only in the more superficial fibers. The superficial fibers are large and soft, but they grow smaller and harder as they approach the center of the lens; this difference becomes more marked as life advances, so much so that the central part appears homogeneous. This has led to the division of the lens into two parts, called respectively nucleus and cortex, although the hardened lens can be divided into innumerable layers, which show a tendency to break into sectors, the division taking place at the radiating lines already mentioned. The substance of the lens is covered by a thin elastic membrane, which is divided into two parts, called the anterior and posterior capsule. The anterior capsule is the thicker and stronger of the two, its center being its thickest part, while the center of the posterior capsule is its thinnest part. Covering the entire anterior surface of the lens substance is a single layer of nucleated cells; these are the formative cells of the lens; near the periphery of the lens, fibers may be seen growing from them; they are attached to the posterior surface of the anterior capsule and also to the lens tissue by a layer of cement substance. There are no cells between the posterior capsule and the lens tissue. The lens is held in place by the suspensory ligament, called the zonule of Zinn. This membranous ligament is a continuation of the hyaloid membrane of the vitreous, which, at the ora serrata, splits into two sheets, the outer one of which becomes fibrous in character and is closely attached to the pars ciliaris retina, being more firmly attached to the convex surfaces of the ciliary folds than to the depressions. At the thickest part of the ciliary body, this membrane breaks up into bundles of fibres, some of which become adherent to the anterior capsule, some to the margin of the lens sac and some extend a short distance upon the posterior lens capsule. A saculated circular space found around the lens and within the zonule of Zinn is called the canal of Petit. The function of the lens is to refract the rays of light that go to form ocular images; also, to vary the refractive power of the eye. Accommodation is the term applied to this power of varying the refraction of the eye. It is brought about by the inherent elasticity of the lens, the contraction of the ciliary muscle and the elasticity of the zonule of Zinn. Relieved of all tension, the tendency of the lens is to become more convex; during life this tendency is restrained by the elastic tension of the ligament of Zinn, its tension being dependent upon the intra-ocular tension and the state of the ciliary muscle, contraction of this muscle reducing the tension of the zonule, so allowing the lens to increase its convexity. The lens and its capsule contain no blood-vessels, its nutrition being maintained by fluid from the ciliary body.

The Vitreous.

The vitreous is a beautiful, transparent, jelly-like substance, filling that part of the eyeball which lies posterior to the lens. It is covered by a delicate transparent membrane, called the hyaloid membrane, and is pierced by the hyaloid canal, which extends from the optic disk to the region of the posterior capsule; this canal is about 2 mm. in diameter, and in foetal life the hyaloid artery passes through it. It forms one of the lymph canals of the eye, and contains a watery fluid and some fibrous tissue, and is lined by a delicate membrane. Other lymph canals are found near the surface of the vitreous. Although analysis shows the vitreous to contain 98.6 parts water, the slight amount of solid matter it contains is enough to give it a semi-solid consistency. It belongs to the connective tissue group of substances. Within it are found wandering cells, also delicate fibers of connective tissue cells, some of which are supposed to be the remains of minute arteries which penetrate the vitreous during fcetal life, while others are given off from the hyaloid membrane at the ora serrata. The vitreous forms part of the refractive system of the eye. Its nutrition is maintained by a nutrient fluid given off by the vessels of the ciliary body, choroid and retina.

The Choroid.

The choroid is situated between the retina and sclerotic, and extends from the ora serrata to the optic nerve entrance. It is essentially a vascular structure, being made up of arteries, veins and capillaries. Between the meshes of the arteries and veins are found connective tissues, pigmented and non-pigmented connective tissue cells. Between the capillaries no pigment is found, but a soft transparent substance permeates the capillary meshes, which are finer here than in any other part of the body. At the fovea centralis the capillary layer is thicker and its meshes finer than in any other part of the choroid. The various vascular structures of the choroid form such well de-fined lamina that it is often described as being divided into three layers: (1) the layer of large vessels which is the most external, and consists largely of veins; (2) the layer of medium-sized vessels, which is the middle layer; and (3) the layer of capillaries, which is the most internal of the three, being sep-arated from the retina by a thin hyaline membrane called the lamina vitrea. The suprachoroid, a loose, fibrous, pigmented structure, joins the choroid at the sclerotic. The arteries of the choroid are derived from the short posterior ciliary, which pierces the sclerotic around the optic nerve entrance. The veins converge, in the form of whorls, to four or five main trunks, called the venae vorticosoe, which pierce the sclerotic very obliquely a short distance behind the equator of the eyeball. The nerves are derived from the ciliary, and are distributed to the blood-vessels, among which ganglionic cells are found. The choroid is not a sensitive membrane; destructive changes often take place in it without causing any pain. Lymphatic canals and spaces are found around the blood vessels and between the various layers. The function of the choroid is to nourish the posterior layers of the retina, although that part which surrounds the ora serrata may assist in maintaining the nutrition of the vitreous.

The Retina.

The retina proper, or optical part, extends from the optic nerve entrance to the junction of the choroid with the ciliary body, ending in an irregular dentated border, termed the ora serrata. The pigment layer and a certain portion of the supporting tissue elements of the retina extend over the ciliary body to the base of the iris, this part of the membrane being called the pars ciliaris retinae. A layer of retinal pigment and connective tissue lines the pos-terior surface of the iris and extends to its periphery. The structure of the retina proper is very complicated, and has been studied with great minute-ness by anatomists. For our purpose, it will serve to consider it as made up of percipient, nervous and supporting elements, and a layer of pigment cells. The pigment layer is the most external, and lies nearest the choroid. Next come the percipient elements, which are generally described as consisting of two layers, the most external one being called the layer of rods and cones, the other one being called the nuclear or granular layer; but the elements of this latter layer are simply the nuclei of the rods and cones. The relative number of the rods and cones differ in different parts of the retina; near the ora serrata the rods greatly predominate; near the central part a single cone will be surrounded by several rows of rods; still nearer there will be found only a single circle of rods around a cone, and in the macula lutea, which is an irregular, oval-shaped spot of yellow color situated in the central part of the retina, only cones are found. The diameter of the macula lutea is about 1.25 mm. In its center is a depression called the fovea centralis, which is the center of visual acuity, the ability to distinguish the form of objects being greater here than at any other part of the retina. The cerebral and nervous elements of the retina consist principally of layers of bipolar and multipolar cells, and the layer of rods and cones. The nuclei of the rods and cones give off processes which terminate in numerous fine filaments, which interlace with those given off by the multipolar ganglionic cells. The multipolar cells terminate in an axis cylinder, which is continued to the brain as a nerve fiber of the optic nerve. A point to be remembered is that there is no direct anatomical continuity between the several elements. The supporting tissue of the retina is termed the sustentacular tissue or fibers of Müller. These fibers serve the purpose of connective tissue, passing between the nerve elements in the form of delicate radial fibers, containing nuclei, and giving off delicate fibrillse laterally. Between the layer of nerve fibers and the next layer the ends of the fibers coalesce, forming the internal limiting membrane of the retina. Near the inner termination of the body of the rods and cones the radial fibers also coalesce, forming the external limiting membrane of the retina. Towards the ora serrata the Müllerine fibers are well developed and very numerous, while at the macula they are very delicate and few in number. The retinal vessels consist of the central artery and vein. The artery is a branch of the ophthalmic; it pierces the optic nerve about 20 mm. behind the eyeball and passes through the optic disk at about its center, where it divides into a superior and inferior branch; these again divide and subdivide and curve around the macula lutea, sending fine branches to it, but none reach the center of the fovea. The branches of the central artery do not anastomose with each other. Some fine branches given off at the optic disk anastomose with the choroidal arteries, this being the only place in the eye where the retinal and ciliary systems unite. The retinal vein and its branches accompany the central artery. The lymph canals follow the blood-vessels, and the lymph escapes through the optic disk. The capillaries of the central artery do not extend beyond the inner nuclear layer, the external layers of the retina deriving their nutrition from the capillary layer of the choroid. All parts of the living retina, with the exception of the pigment layer and the blood contained within the vessels, are transparent. The retina rapidly becomes opaque in disease and after death. The function of the retina is to receive rays of light and convert them into a form of energy capable of being transmitted to the brain.

The Optic Nerve.

The optic nerve is made up of retinal nerve fibers; they pass from the eye through the lamina cribrosa. The lamina cribrosa is made up principally of fibers from the choroid and the internal third of the sclera. The outer two-thirds of the sclera go to form the outer sheath of the optic nerve, which is continuous with the dura mater of the brain, and it is called the dural sheath. Two other membranes are found; the most internal, called the pial sheath, is a continuation of the pia mater of the brain; it forms the vascular and supporting sheath of the optic nerve; it is closely in contact with the optic nerve, and sends numerous fine prolongations between the nerve fibres, forming a supporting network. Its arteries are derived from the anterior cerebral. The middle sheath is derived from the arachnoid membrane. Between this sheath and the outer ones are two lymph spaces, one being termed the subdural and the other the subarachnoidal; they are continuous with the cerebral lymph spaces. The fibers of the optic nerve pass to nearly all parts of the brain, but the fibers that go to the nuclei of the third nerve and those that go to the cortex of the occipital lobes are of the greatest interest to the oculist. It will simplify the understanding of diseases of the optic nerve to consider it as divided into three portions: (1) The intra-ocular portion, viz., that part of the nerve which is contained within the eyeball and lamina cribrosa. The fibers of this portion have no myaline sheaths, and being constricted by the lamina cribrosa they are particularly liable to disease. (2) The retro-ocular or intra-orbital portion which extends from the eyeball to the optic foramen. This portion of the nerve is longer than the distance from the eyeball to the optic foramen, and, as a consequence, it is thrown into two folds bearing some resemblance to the letter S. This arrangement allows of great mobility of the eyeball without stretching the nerve. The part of the nerve within the optic foramen is very much prone to disease. (3) That part which lies within the cranial cavity, and which is divided into the nerve proper, which is very short, the optic chiasm and the optic tract. The optic chiasm is formed by the crossing of some of the fibers of the two optic nerves. The fibers from the temporal half of each eye cross over and join the fibers of the temporal half of the opposite eye, thus forming the tract. In this way the fibers from the left half of each eye form the right optic tract and go to the right side of the brain. Fibers from each of the macula lutea are found in both optic tracts. Fully one-third of the fibers of the optic nerve come from the macular region; they are termed the papillomacular fibers. The part of the nerve which lies within the cranial cavity is covered only by the pial sheath, the other two sheaths becoming continuous with the membranes of the brain at the optic foramen. The function of the optic nerve is to convey retinal impressions to the brain.

Chapter Seven - Optical Principles Governing Vision

For the purpose of studying the physiology of vision, a human eye may be divided into three parts, the first being the collecting or refracting portion, consisting of the cornea, aqueous humor, crystalline lens and vitreous. These are called the dioptric or refracting media. The second is the receiving and transforming portion, and it consists of the retina. The third being the transmitting portion consists of the optic nerve. A brief consideration of a few optical laws will facility our study. Light may be considered as a form of energy generated by luminous bodies; this energy travels in wave-like motions, in a substance termed luminous ether, which is supposed to pervade all space. Luminous bodies are made up of a collection of luminous points — a luminous point being a center from which rays of light emanate. A ray of light is a line along which light is transmitted. Rays of light are never curved; those that diverge from their source are called diverging rays, those that converge are called converging rays and those that seem to issue parallel are termed parallel rays. A pencil of rays is a collection of rays that seem to have a common center. A body that allows rays of light to pass freely through it is said to be transparent. A body that checks their passage is termed opaque. It must be understood that these terms are only relative, no substance being absolutely transparent or opaque. Absorption, reflection and refraction are terms that are applied to the behavior of light rays when they impinge upon certain bodies. Absorption means the conversion of light into some other form of energy, generally heat; this is usually a property of dark opaque bodies with irregular surfaces, such as black velvet, lamp black, etc. Reflection means a bending back of the impinging rays of light into the medium from whence they came. Light colored bodies, with highly polished surfaces, make the best reflectors. Reflection is divided into regular and irregular. After regular reflection the character of the ray of light is not changed. Diverging, converging and parallel rays are reflected as diverging, converging and parallel rays. Irregularly reflecting surfaces change the character of the rays impinging upon them, the rays after reflection issuing as if generated within the reflecting body, and their degree of divergence will depend upon the distance of the reflecting body from the observer and not upon the kind of incident rays. This property of irregular reflection is of great importance, as by it nonluminous bodies are made visible. Rays from regular reflectors simply give the image of the source of the light. An illuminated body is one that is made visible by reflected or transmitted light. Refraction is the bending of the rays of light that pass from one medium into another; it takes place at the surface of division It is the property of transparent bodies, whose power of retarding light differs from that of the medium, in which the light is incident and in which the dividing surfaces of the two media are not parallel. If rays of light strike a plane reflecting surface perpendicularly they are reflected back upon themselves. If the incident ray forms an angle with a line drawn perpendicular to a regular reflecting surface, the reflected ray will form an angle with this perpendicular line equal to the angle formed by the incident ray. This is the law of regular reflection, viz.: The angle of reflection is equal to the angle of incidence, and is in the same plane with it. Mirrors are samples of regular reflectors; they may be of any shape. Plane and concave ones are most commonly used in ophthalmoscopy. Two plane mirrors may be so inclined that the reflected rays from each will cross each other. This point of crossing is called a focus. A concave spherical mirror may be conceived to be made up of an infinite number of minute planes, so inclined that rays after reflection will tend to a focus. The focus for parallel incident rays is the principal focus of the mirror; it is situated on the principal axis, which is a line drawn through the center of the mirror and the center of the sphere of which the concave mirror forms a part. Diverging rays impinging upon a concave mirror will, after reflection, be rendered parallel, converging or less diverging. If they diverge from a point situated at the principal focus of the mirror they will become parallel rays after reflection. If the rays diverge from a point beyond the principal focus, they will converge to a focus after reflection; and the further the point of incidence is from the mirror, the nearer will be the focus of convergence. The foci for rays other than parallel are called secondary foci. The point of incidence and the point of union are conjugate foci. Rays incident within the principal focus will, after reflection, still be diverging, though less so than before reflection; and the nearer the mirror to the point of incidence, the more diverging will be the reflected rays. If they be retraced, a point will be found from which they seem to proceed, and this point is called a negative or virtual focus. Refraction may be divided into regular and irregular. Regular refraction is produced by homogeneous, transparent bodies bounded by regular surfaces. Irregular refraction is produced by bodies whose structure is of unequal refractive power, or whose surfaces are irregular. The laws governing regular refraction have been formulated, but not those governing irregular refraction. Rays of light passing from one medium to another of different density, will not be refracted if they strike the second medium perpendicularly to its surface, though their motion may be retarded or accelerated, depending upon the relative density of the two media. If the second medium is more dense or more highly refractive than the first, the light will be retarded in passing through it; if less dense, it will be accelerated. If the incident rays form an angle with the perpendicular, and the second medium is more dense than the first, the refracted rays will be bent towards the perpendicular; if the second medium is less dense, the refracted rays will be bent from the perpendicular. Upon these facts is founded the first law of regular refraction, viz: Rays of light in passing from a rare to a dense medium are bent towards the perpendicular. And, conversely, rays of light in passing from a dense to a rare medium are bent from the perpendicular. The term "dense medium" maybe used as being synomyinous with the term "more refracting medium," although some substances are exceptions to this rule, they being less dense, but more highly refracting than others. Measurements of the sines of the angles of incidence and refraction in a given medium have shown that they bear a constant ratio, no matter how great or how small the angle of incidence may be, if the second medium is of greater density than the first, or incident, medium. For example, in the case of glass and air, the sine of the angle of incidence, or the angle in air, should bear to the sine of the angle of refraction, or the angle in glass, the ratio of 3 to 2. From these data Snell evolved the second law of refraction, or the law of sines, viz.: The sine of the angle of incidence has to sine of the angle of refraction always the same ratio for the same medium. It is to be remembered that Snell's law is only applicable to homogeneous substances. The number which expresses the ratio of the sine of the angle of incidence to the sine of the angle of refraction is called the Index of Refraction. This is, in the case of air and glass, 3/2, or, as it is most always expressed, 1.50. In the case of air and water, it is 1.333. The number which expresses the index of refraction of a given substance is used as an index of the refractive power of that substance, for the index of refraction increases with the refractive power. In the case of a plate of glass with plane parallel surfaces, parallel incident rays impinging at an angle will, after refraction, issue as parallel rays, but they will be displaced laterally; the greater the thickness of the glass, the greater will be this lateral displacement. A transparent body, in the form of a wedge, will constitute a prism. If the prism be made of glass, or any other transparent substance whose index of refraction is greater than air, it will bend all rays of light, through its inclined surfaces, towards its base. If two prisms are placed base to base they will constitute the most elementary form of a converging lens. It will be a converging lens, because it will cause all rays of light refracted by it to converge, each of the prisms bending the rays towards their common base. If the prisms were placed apex to apex they would form a diverging lens. If the rays of light from a given source were limited to two, and if they were incident, one upon each of the prisms forming the converging lens, they would, after refraction, cross each other, and their point of crossing or union would be a focus. It would be what is known in optics as a real focus. In the case of the diverging lens there would be no real focus, but if the refracted rays were retraced, a point would be found where they would cross, and this point would be known as a virtual focus, sometimes called negative or imaginary. If the incident light consisted of a number of rays they would cross after refraction by the converging lens and form a more or less perfect line, whose direction would be parallel with the base line of the prisms forming the lens. This line is called a focal line. In considering the behavior of light incident in the more refracting medium, we find that, in order to be refracted, the incident ray must form an angle within certain limits which differ in different substances. This angle is called the critical angle. In the case of glass and air — the ray being incident in the glass — the critical angle is 40°. If the incident angle exceeded that figure, the light would not escape from the glass but would be reflected at the surface of the two media, back into the first, and follow the law of regular reflection. Reflection under such conditions is termed total reflection. If the angle of a prism is greater than twice the critical angle of its substance, light will not be refracted by it, but will be reflected. Such prisms are called reflecting prisms. They are used in binocular ophthalmoscopes, microscopes, etc. The angle formed by the two refracting surfaces of a prism is called its refracting angle. Lenses used in ophthalmoscopic practice are transparent bodies, bounded by spherical or cylindrical surfaces. They are generally made of glass or rock crystal. Lenses are divided into two main classes; those that converge rays of light, and those that diverge them. The first are termed converging, convex or plus lenses, and are designated by the plus (+) sign. Those of the second class are termed diverging, concave or minus lenses, and are designated by the minus (—) sign. A body of greater refracting power than air, bounded by spherical surfaces, would have the property of causing all rays refracted by it to be bent towards a common center. The rays would cross at this center and then diverge. The place of crossing or union would be termed a focus. A line perpendicular to the center of the refracting surface and passing through the refracting body would be the principal axis of the lens. Lines directed to the center of the sphere of which this surface forms a part, cutting its surface at a part other than its center, would be called secondary axes. Rays of light occupying the place of these lines would be called axial rays, and, being perpendicular to the refracting surface, they would not be refracted. Incident rays parallel with the principal axis would be brought to a focus on it; this focus would be the principal focus of the lens. The foci of converging or diverging rays would be secondary foci. Rays parallel with the secondary axes would be brought to focus on them; these foci would be the principal foci of the secondary axes. The point from which rays of light emanate, as well as the point from which they converge, are both called foci, one being the focus of incidence and the other the focus of refraction. The surface separating two media of different refracting power is termed a refracting surface.

The medium through which the light passes before impinging upon the refracting surface is called the first medium. The second medium is the medium into which the light enters after passing through the refracting surface. Bear in mind that the bending, or refracting, of a ray takes place at the refracting surface. The first principal focus is the focus for rays parallel in the second medium. The second principal focus would be situated in the second medium, at such a distance from the dividing surface that the rays after passing this surface would be parallel to the principal axis in the first medium. These two foci are called cardinal points. There are two other cardinal points in a simple refracting system, viz., the principal point and the nodal point. The principal point is a point on the principal axis where the refracting surface cuts it. The nodal point is a point on the principal axis where the secondary axes cross it and each other.

To recapitulate, the cardinal points of a single refracting surface separating two media are four in number, as follows:

The principal point.
The first principal focus.
The second principal focus.
The nodal point.

A plane drawn through the principal point at right angles to the principal axis would be called the principal plane. Planes drawn at right angles to the principal foci would be the first and second principal focal planes. The principal axis is also known as the optic axis. Conjugate foci are foci that have a definite relation to each other. For example, if light is diverging from a focus, and after refraction is brought to a focus, the position of one focus will influence the position of the other. If one is brought near the line the other will recede, and vice versa. Spherical converging lenses are of three kinds — planoconvex, in which one surface is convex and the other plane; biconvex, in which both surfaces are convex; meniscus, in which one surface is convex and the other concave — the convex surface being the stronger of the two. Spherical diverging lenses are also of three kinds — the plano-concave, the biconcave, the concavo-convex. In the last named the concave surface is stronger than the convex surface. Spherical lenses may be considered to be made up of the sections of a sphere. We estimate the curvature of the lens by the length of the radius of curvature of each surface. The radius of curvature is half the diameter of the sphere of which the lens forms a part. The shorter the radius of curvature, the more powerful the lens of a given index of refraction. The radius of curvature and the index of refraction are the two factors required in estimating the strength of a lens. Spherical lenses are distinguished from cylindrical lenses, in that they either bring rays of light to a focus or cause them to diverge as if they proceeded from a focus, the first being an example of a plus lens and the second being an example of a minus lens. A cylindrical lens, being a sector of a cylinder, refracts only the rays that strike it at right angles to its length. The length of such a lens is in the direction of the length of the cylinder of which it forms a part. A central line coinciding with the direction of the cylinder is called the axis of the cylindrical lens. Plus cylindrical lenses form sections of a solid cylinder, being bounded on one side by a cylindrical surface and on the other by a plane surface. Minus cylindrical lenses form sections of a body whose inner surface is cylindrical and whose outer surface is plane. The above described lenses tend to bring rays of light towards, or diverge them from, a line. The direction of this line coincides with the axis of the lens. When we speak of spherical and cylindrical lenses bringing rays to a point or line, we must not be understood to mean a mathematical point or line. The curve of such lenses is such that raws of light striking it near the periphery are more refracted than those striking near the center. As a consequence, there are many points between the focus for the central rays and the focus for the marginal rays. The stronger and larger the lens the greater would be this wandering from a true focus. This is called spherical aberration. Only in weak lenses, or in those in which only the central part is made use of, can the spherical aberration be ignored. It is corrected in most optical instruments by making use ot several weak lenses in place of one strong one, and by varying the curve and the material, and by the use of diaphragms — that is, screens which limit the path of light to certain parts of the lens. Chromatic aberration is another factor that must be recognized when making use of strong lenses or prisms; it is due to the compound nature of light. A beam of white light is made up of rays of unequal wave lengths and velocities. A beam of white light refracted by a strong prism will present a band of colors if the refracted rays be received upon a screen. This color band is termed the solar spectrum. While the spectrum is doubtless made up of innumerable colors which invisibly merge into each other, seven colors have been named, and the spectrum is spoken of as consisting of red, orange, yellow, green, blue, indigo and violet. The majority of persons see only six colors in the spectrum. The color-rays are refracted in the order named, the violet being refracted the most and the red rays the least. As a consequence of this difference in refractibility, the violet rays are brought to a focus nearest the lens, the red rays furthest from it, and the other between in the order named. This dispersion can be corrected in a great measure by combining plus and minus lenses of different refracting substances, some refracting substances having relatively greater dispersive power than others. For example, a plus lens of crown glass may be combined with a minus lens of flint glass, the dispersive power of flint glass being much greater than that of crown glass, though its refractive power is but slightly in excess. Lenses in which the chromatic aberration is corrected are called achromatic.

The Formation of Optical Images.

A ray of light given off from a luminous point may be considered as an extension of that point. If the ray be intersected, an image of the point will be found at the place of intersection. The image may or may not be visible, its visibility depending upon a variety of conditions; for example, a sufficient amount of light must be transmitted from the image to make an impression upon the visual organ of the observer, and the image must not be obscured by the overlapping of other images. By a simple experiment, an image of any luminous or illuminated point may be displayed to view. Rays of light from any luminous or illuminated object may be admitted through a small opening into a dark room, and a screen placed so as to receive them. If the opening were of such a size that it would admit only one ray from each of the radiating points of the object, a sharp, clear image would be formed on the screen. This image would be inverted and very much dimmer than the object. If the screen were nearer the opening than the object, the image would be smaller, and the nearer the opening was brought the smaller would be the image; it would be more brightly illuminated because the same number of rays would be received on a smaller surface than when the screen was further from the opening. If the image and the object were an equal distance from the opening, the image and object would be of the same size. If the screen were further from the opening than object, the image would be larger but very dim. In no way in this experiment could the image be made as bright as the object and yet preserve the sharpness of clear definition. By making the opening larger a greater number of rays would be admitted; they would, of course, make the image brighter, but its outlines would be dimmed and rendered indistinct by the overlapping of images formed by the excess of rays admitted, no two rays from one point would strike the screen at the same place on account of their divergence. The reason that the image is inverted relatively to the object is, that rays from the top of the object, in order to enter the opening, are directed downward, and rays from the bottom are directed upward, and they cross each other at the opening; the rays from the upper part of the object going to the lower part of the screen, and the rays from the lower part of the object going to the upper part of the screen. The same would be true of rays from all parts of the object except those from that part opposite the center of the opening. From this experiment we may learn several things of great value in studying the art of using the ophthalmoscope, and of correcting the errors of refraction and accommodation. First, that the rays of light form the image. Second, the nearer the image to the opening or crossing of the rays, the brighter and smaller it will be. Third, that while enlarging the opening increases the illumination it blurs the image. Fourth, that images of objects are inverted relatively to the object. The two principal means of projecting images in ophthalmoscopic practice are convex lenses and concave mirrors. By the use of these instruments, brightly illuminated, sharp images can be obtained, and under certain conditions the image can be made brighter than the object. The part taken by lenses and mirrors in the formation of images can be likened to that of the small opening, with the additional power of collecting a large number of rays diverging from a point in the object and of bringing them to a point in the image. The image formed by a lens is formed on the side opposite the object. An image formed by a mirror is on the same side as the object. The image is projected by refraction in the case of the lens, and by reflection in the case of the mirror. If the object were at an infinite distance, the rays from it would be parallel, and its image would be at the principal focus of the lens and would be very bright and very small. If the object were at the principal focus of the lens, the rays issuing from it would be very divergent, and its image would be at infinity and infinitely large. The same would be true in the case of a concave mirror. If the object were at twice the distance of the principal focus of the lens, its image would be formed at the same distance on the other side of the lens, and would be of the same size. It would not be as brightly illuminated as the object, for the reason that all the rays coming from the object and incident upon the lens would not pass through it, a certain number being lost by reflection from the surface of the lens, while certain others would be absorbed. The fact to be remembered is, that the nearer the object is to the focus of the lens the larger will be the image, and the further from the focus the smaller it will be. If the object were between the focus and the lens, the rays, after passing through the lens, would issue as diverging rays and no real image would be projected. But if the refracted rays were retraced they would seem to unite on the same side of the lens as the object, there forming a collection of negative or virtual foci, termed a virtual image, which would be erect and larger than the object. The point of interest about virtual images is that rays of light that seem to come from them, under the conditions given above, will, if received by an eye, form an image of the object upon the retina, as though the object were situated at the place of the virtual image and were of the same size. If the rays that go to form the lenticular image be traced, their course will be found to be as follows: From the object are given off certain rays that strike the surface of the lens in the direction of its radius of curvature; as a consequence they are perpendicular to that part of the surface which they strike. They undergo no refraction, but cross at the nodal point of the lens. They are called rays of direction or axial rays. All of them, except the one coinciding with its principal axis, are called secondary axes. These secondary axes correspond to the rays that formed the image in the experiments made with the dark room and the small opening. From every point from which are given off axial rays a great number of other rays diverge; these form a cone around each axial ray, the base of which is the lens and the apex of which is the point in the object from which they come. The sum of all these foci form the image of the object. Its place, size, brightness and definition are governed by the same condition as is the principal focus of the lens. An optical image may be formed in the air, in which case it would be called an aerial image. If this image be received upon a screen that does not coincide with the place where the rays forming the image are focused, the image will be blurred and indistinct, and instead of being made up of foci it will be formed of circles of dispersion.

Chapter Eight - Physiology of Vision

The function of the visual organs may be considered under three divisions: (1) That of focusing images; (2) that of receiving, transforming and transmitting the impressions made by the images; (3) that of fusing the two retinal images and interpreting them as a single impression. That part of the eye which focuses the ocular images is called the refractive or dioptric media. It consists of the cornea, aqueous humor, crystalline lens and vitreous humor. These are bounded by refracting surfaces on which the bending of the rays of light takes place. The anterior surface of the cornea is the most important of the refracting surfaces, on account of its separating two media (air and corneal tissue), which differ greatly in refractive power. On account of the surfaces of the cornea being nearly parallel to each other, and on account of the index of refraction of the aqueous humor and the tissue of the cornea differiug but slightly, the cornea is considered as one refracting media bounded by one surface, its anterior one. The cornea acts as a convex lens, and its radius of curvature is about 8 mm. The crystalline is the next most important media; it is a biconvex body, the radius of its anterior surface being 10 mm. and the radius of its posterior surface being 6 mm. when at rest. It is most beautifully adapted to its purpose. The index of refraction of its structure increases from its surface to its center, which is occupied by a dense material called the nucleus, which in a healthy lens is almost spherical in shape. The layers of tissue surrounding this central portion, and which constitutes the rest of the lens, are termed the cortex or cortical part of the lens. The layer-like structure of the lens may be demonstrated by means of a boiled lens; layer after layer may be stripped off, in much the same manner that an onion can be reduced to layers. This peculiar structure increases its refractive power by practically reducing its radius of curvature. The cortical layers act as weak diverging lenses surrounding a very strong converging lens — the nucleus. Chromatic and spherical aberration are also corrected in a great measure by this construction of the lens. The vitreous extends from the lens to the retina; its anterior surface is applied to the posterior surface of the lens, and is concave and of the same radius of curvature; its posterior surface is convex and follows the curve of the retina. The vitreous forms a weak diverging lens. The dioptric apparatus of the eye, as a whole, forms a compound optical instrument acting as a converging lens, the principal focus of which would be, in the case of an emmetropic or normal eye, 22.23 mm behind the center of the cornea. The iris acts as a diaphragm to the refracting apparatus of the eye by regulating the amount of light admitted to the eye. It also, by its contraction, limits the passage of the rays of light to the more central portions of the dioptric apparatus, thus serving to reduce aberration of the rays after refraction. For the purpose of clinical calculation the human eye may, without sensible error, be considered as consisting of a single surface of refraction, whose radius of curvature is 5 mm., and of a single medium, whose index of refraction is 4/3. Such an eye would have a posterior focus of 20 mm., its nodal point would be 5 mm. from the center of the cornea and 15 mm. from the retina, and its anterior focus would be 15 mm. from the center of the cornea. The reductions here given were suggested by Donders, and such a diagrammatic eye is known as "the reduced eye of Donders." It is of very great value in calculating the size of retinal images of external objects; also of the circles of diffusion in refractive and accommodative errors. Light striking the anterior surface of the cornea is caused to converge; this converging pencil of rays passes through the pupil, impinges upon the lens, undergoes refraction by its several layers and nucleus, and, being made more convergent, it passes through the vitreous, and, if the retina is at the place of focus, an image of the object will be formed upon it. If the retina is not at this position, but in front or behind the place where the image is formed, it would receive, instead of an assemblage of points of light, numerous overlapping images of the points of the object. These blurred images are called circles of diffusion. If the retina were in front of the posterior focus of the refracting apparatus, it would receive the circles of diffusion before the rays had come to a focus; if behind the place of focus, it would receive the diffusion circles which are formed after the rays of light have come to a focus and crossed. In either case the retinal image would lack definition, and the object would appear indistinct and blurred. The greater the circles of diffusion the greater the blurring. The ocular image may be indistinct on account of imperfections of the refracting structure. The surfaces may not be true, the radius of curvature of one meridian differing from that of another, or the individual meridians may be irregular, or there may be opacities in any of the media, either fixed or floating, or a difference in the indices of refraction of different sectors of any of the refracting media may exist. Any of these imperfections will cause lack of distinctness of outline of the ocular images. The function of the retina is to receive ocular images and transform that form of motion known as light into a form of motion that can be conveyed to the brain by the nervous structure of the retina, the optic nerve and ganglia. A line drawn through the nodal point to the fovea centralis of the retina is called the visual line; it forms a small angle with the optic axis. The fovea is the most sensitive part of the retina for form sense. The function of monocular vision depends upon the integrity of all the above-named structures. Binocular vision, or single vision with both eyes, is dependent upon functional perfection of the structures already mentioned, and upon the function of fusion being intact, and this depends upon the functional integrity of many structures, the most important being the recti and oblique muscles. The function termed accommodation is the power that the eye has of changing the direction of rays of light that pass through the lens. By it the eve can focus rays coining from distant or near-by objects. As an object is brought near the eye, the divergence of the rays coming from it increases. Under such conditions, if the place where the rays are focused is fixed, the power of the refractive part of the eye will have to be increased. This is the condition in the human eye, and the change in refractive power is brought about by the contraction of the ciliary muscle; this contraction relaxes the zonule of Zinn, which allows the lens to become more convex by its own elasticity. This function is more active in youth. Examination of great numbers of eyes has shown that this power declines from the age of ten years, and, of course, as the power of accommodation declines the near point recedes. When it has receded to eight inches, the term presbyopia is used to express the condition. The term Refraction is used to indicate the power of the refractive media of an eye when its ciliary muscle is at rest;

it expresses the minimum refractive power of the eye. The term Accommodation means the dynamic refraction, or the power which the eye has of changing its refractive state. The term Emmetropia is applied to an eye adapted to parallel rays of light — *i.e.,* an emmetropic eye brings parallel rays of light to g focus upon its retina without exercising its power of accommodation. Ametropia is a term applied to an eye in which the refraction varies from that of an emmetropic eye.

Chapter Nine - The Study of The Normal Fundus and the Art of Using the Ophthalmoscope

The Ophthalmoscope was invented by Helmholtz in 1851. Its invention placed ophthalmoscopy upon a scientific basis. Formerly it was supposed that all rays of light entering the eye were absorbed by the retinal and choroidal pigment, and that therefore none would be reflected by its fundus. This was proved to be a false idea by several investigators, who had observed that the eyes of certain animals would glow in a darkened room, but not in absolute darkness, thus showing that the light came from some external source, and that the glow was due to reflection from the fundus of the eye.

Other observers had been able to see the retinal vessels of a cat's eye by holding it under water, and a reflex from the fundus of the human eye had been seen in the case of a person whose iris had been torn off. Helmholtz, having a great knowledge of optics, and being familiar with the anatomy of the eye, was able to make use of these observations; and he discovered that the reason that we cannot ordinarily see the fundus of the eye is on account of its optical construction, it being the property of the human eye, in common with other compound optical instruments, to cause the rays of light which emerge from it to follow the path of incidence. The diameter of the pupil determines the diameter of the cones of rays received on the fundus. It also limits the path of the rays to the central part of the refracting media, and restricts the emergent rays to the same narrow course. In emmetropia the diameter of the reflected bundle of rays depends entirely upon the size of the pupil, the size of the emergent bundle of rays in ametropia being influenced to a much less extent by the state of the pupil. The fundus of the human eye, being an irregular reflecting surface, has the property of causing rays of light reflected by it to diverge from its surface as if they were generated within it. Parallel, diverging and converging incident rays all become diverging rays after reflection by the fundus. Upon refraction by the refractive media, they emerge from the eye as parallel, diverging or converging rays, depending upon the dioptric power of the eye. A pencil of diverging rays, passing through the pupil and directed towards the source of illumination, would form a larger surface of light than a pencil of parallel or converging rays. If the observer could place his eye sufficiently near the flame he might receive some of those diverging rays upon his retina; he would then see a portion of the fundus undergoing examination. If the observer could place his eye at the source of illumination, he would be able to see the fundus of the eye, even if the pupil were small and its refraction emmetropic. This might be accomplished in various ways, either by placing in the flame a tube with a screen attached to protect the observer's eye, or by changing the direction of the incident rays by means of a mirror. Helmholtz chose the latter way when constructing his first ophthalmoscope. It consisted of three parallel plane glass plates, set at an angle of 56°, and held so as to, reflect the light into the patient's eye.

This construction of the instrument polarized the light by reflection, thus doing away, to a great extent, with the annoying reflection from the center of the cornea. The observer looked obliquely through plates which were fixed in a triangular box, the plates forming the hypothenuse. The smaller perpendicular surface of this box was perforated and opened into a cup-shaped addition which enclosed the eye of the observer. Although this instrument gave a very feeble illumination, with it Helmholtz and Von Graefe examined a great many eyes, and determined their refraction by the aid of several pairs of concave and convex spectacles, and even measured the dioptric power of dead eyes.

The use of the convex object lens, held between the ophthalmoscope and the eye of the patient, was a later discovery, and gave rise to "indirect ophthalmoscopy." The ophthalmoscope has been modified and improved by numerous inventors. The kind of an ophthalmoscope to be preferred will depend upon the use one intends to make of it. If for direct examination, one with a small concave mirror of short focus (8 mm.), having a central perforation not larger than 2 ½ mm. in diameter, should be chosen, because only that part of the mirror which immediately surrounds the aperture is available in the direct examination, and should the sight-hole be larger than the pupil the fundus could not be satisfactorily illuminated. It should be capable of being tilted about 25°, independent of the disk which contains the correcting lenses. This disk is placed behind the mirror, and arranged to rotate in such a manner that the lenses are brought successively behind the sighthole of the mirror. The lenses should center, that is, the centers of the lenses should coincide with the center of the sight-hole, and every good ophthalmoscope has an arrangement for this purpose. The lenses should have a diameter of not less than 6 mm., and there should be enough of them to measure the refraction as near as half a dioptre. For the indirect examination should be chosen one with a concave mirror of about 20 cm. focus and 33 mm. diameter, with a sight-hole about three and a-half millimetres in diameter. An instrument of these proportions will give the best results, both in the amount of illumination of the fundus and definition of the image formed on the observer's retina. For this method of examination are required only lenses enough to correct any error of refraction or accommodation existing in the observer's eye, in addition to a convex lens, called "the objective," which is used to form the real image seen in indirect ophthalmoscopy.

A plane mirror is used in skiascopy and in the examination of the vitreous. Some ophthalmoscopes contain all these features, but they are large, heavy and expensive. Loring's latest model is probably the best one for general " use, if only one is to be used. It consists of a concave mirror made of silvered glass, of a focal length of 25 cm., of a height of 33 mm., of a breadth of 19 mm., pierced by an opening 3 mm. in diameter, called the sight-hole; it is swung on two pivots, and is known as the "tilting mirror." At the back of the mirror is a disk containing sixteen lenses and a quadrant containing four lenses, both capable of rotating and centering their lenses. These lenses can be combined, giving a series of lenticular strengths, all that is required in testing refraction. The lenses of this instrument are 6 mm. in diameter. It is well-made and well-balanced. Objective lenses of two and three inch focus accompany it.

To examine the eye by the ophthalmoscope, we must consider the kind of light used and the laws governing light; also, the anatomical, physiological or pathological condition of the eyes of both the examiner and the examined. Either artificial or daylight may be used; the former is to be preferred for general ophthalmoscopy. If daylight is used, diffuse light must be selected, and preferably that which is reflected from a white cloud. Direct sunlight must never be used. The vitreous may be coagulated by the concentration of the sun's rays into the eye by the objective lens of an ophthalmoscope. To make the examination by daylight, a darkened room, with a small opening to admit light, is necessary. The back of the patient being directed a little to one side of the light, the examination proceeds as with artificial light. Of the artificial lights, a lamp or gas bracket with an Argand burner is to be preferred, on account of the large and homogeneous and steady flame with which it burns. The lamp light is the steadier of the two, but its position is not so easily changed, which must be done during the various stages of the examination. Electric light is objectionable on account of the small luminous surface it presents, and in the case of the arc light of its disagreeable flickering. Lights such as the Welsbach, in which a fibrous network is heated to incandescence, are not to be recommended, because the network, being pictured on the fundus, interferes with the clearness of the ophthalmoscopic image. A candle is of service when the examination must be made at the bedside.

The optical laws which have to be considered are those that govern regular refraction from spherical and plane surfaces and those which govern regular refraction from spherical lenses, with special reference to the law of conjugate foci. The point from which incident rays of light diverge and the point to which refracted rays converge are conjugate foci. If the incident focus is brought towards the lens, the refracted focus will recede, and vice versa. The position of one is dependent upon the other. In indirect ophthalmoscopy, the real image is formed by the objective lens. This image and that portion of the fundus of which it is the image are conjugate foci. Or, to speak more strictly, a single luminous point and its retinal image are conjugate foci. The most noticeable object found in the fundus of the eye on ophthalmoscopic examination is the optic nerve entrance, termed the optic disk, or the optical papilla. It appears as a round or oval disk, or spot, of a pale pinkish gray tint, but variegated in structure and color. The disk is a true papilla, especially towards the nasal side, but it appears to be in the plane of the choroid; this is due to the transparency of the optic nerve fibers. The white surface of the disk is due to the lamina cribrosa. The gray medullary sheaths being given off at different planes in the lamina cribrosa gives rise to the gray mottled appearance observed in some disks. Its pink color is due to its vascularity, the nasal side being the most vascular. By contrast, the temporal side sometimes appears very white. The color of the disk varies with the quality of the light employed, daylight giving a less vivid and paler line. The same is true of the other parts of the fundus. Gaslight gives a vivid red in the direct examination. With daylight the fundus is a rose-pink color by both methods of examination. The diameter of the optic disk varies from one and two-tenths (1.2) to one and six-tenths (1.6) millimetres. When its contour is oval, the long diameter is usually vertical with the proportion of nine to seven, the average transverse diameter being about one and fourteenths millimetres. The disk is usually closely surrounded by the choroid; when this is not the case, the sclerotic can be seen forming white crescents, or even a white ring, around the disk, giving, at times, the appearance of an ectasia. Crescentic figures of pigment are common at the outer border, sometimes at the inner, rarely found at the upper or lower. A complete ring of pigment is sometimes found. Around the disk is the scleral ring, which is due to the union of the dural and pial sheaths which join the sclerotic at this point. This ring appears whiter and less vascular than the next zone, which is called the vascular zone. Next we find the pars opticus, or clear spot, which is often filled with the connective tissue string, the remains of the fibrous sheath surrounding the central artery. This is generally given up at the pars opticus, and looks like a flat white spot. When this sheath is given up, further back there are found what are called physiological excavations. They appear as funnel-shaped white depressions, which vary greatly in size and depth in normal eyes. In the pars opticus is sometimes found the sheath of the hyaloid artery, which may extend for some distance into the vitreous humor, appearing as an irregular white body projecting above the plane of the fundus. The optic disk is situated about three millimetres from the macula lutea, towards the nasal side, and about one millimetre below the level of a horizontal line drawn through the posterior pole of the eye.

The macula lutea, or yellow spot, including the fovea centralis, is situated in the fundus directly in the line of vision. It is one of the most difficult parts of the fundus to examine when the eye is normal, contraction of the pupil being very marked when light is thrown upon this sensitive part of the fundus. The corneal reflection interferes with a clear view of the central part of the retina when the pupil is small. The macula is elliptical in shape, and is from one to two millimetres in diameter. The retina is thicker near the macula than in any other part of the fundus, being 5 mm. there, while at the ora serrata it is only 1 mm. At the fovea centralis, which is in the center of the macula lutea, it is 2 mm. in thickness. The diameter of the fovea is from 2/10 to 4/10 mm. It contains none of the yellow coloring matter that gives the macula lutea its name. This tint is never seen with the ophthalmoscope. The hyaloid membrane of the vitreous is very thin over the center of the fovea, while behind it the choroid is thickened on account of the great increase of the capillary layer of vessels, which is not only enlarged, but occupies the place of the larger blood-vessels, and even encroaches on the lamina supra choroidea.

Principally on account of the great vascularity of its back ground and its thinness, the fovea is of a brighter hue than the other parts of the retina, although in some cases, where there is a great development of pigment, it will appear as a dark spot l or even quite black. Within a central area, of about 5/10 mm. in diameter, the macula is devoid of blood vessels, although at and around the macula they are very numerous. The retinal and choroidal vessels will demand our attention. The arteries are of a lighter color and generally smaller and less tortuous than the veins. A condition which should always be looked for is the venous pulse which appears at or near the center of the disk, where the veins bend over into the retina, though sometimes it can be seen as far as the edge of the disk. It is seen in the normal eyes, and can be increased by pressure upon the eyeball. The arterial pulse is seen only in diseased eyes.   The refractive index of the walls of the retinal vessels being almost the same as that of the retina, it is very difficult to see them. What is seen in a healthy fundus is the red column of blood which occupies about one-half the diameter of the blood-vessels; the plasma or colorous part of the blood and the walls of the vessels make up the other half. The "light streak," which is of a straw color, and about one-third the diameter of the blood-vessels, is due to the reflection and refraction from the vessels. It should be noted with great attention, for on its clearness and definition we may base our estimation of the refraction and the health of the fundus. The condition of the cornea, lens and vitreous must be determined before attempting to test the refraction of the eye by the ophthalmoscope. The cornea and lens are best examined by what is known as "oblique illumination." This is nothing more than concentrating light on the cornea and crystalline lens by a convex lens held so that its focus strikes their surfaces obliquely. The angle may be varied so that the anterior or posterior, or any part of the cornea, can be brought into view. The same is true of the anterior chamber, the lens and the anterior part of the vitreous humor. It is a very valuable method of examination, and should never be neglected, but should be made before the ophthal-moscopic examination is undertaken. It will disclose very small opacities or irregularities in the above-mentioned structures. In order to correctly esti-mate refraction by direct or indirect ophthalmoscopy, it is necessary to have had considerable experience in ordinary ophthalmoscopy. To make an oph-thalmoscopic examination the patient should be seated in a darkened room. The light should be placed at either his right or left side, depending upon which eye is to be examined. At the right side for the right eye, and at the left side for the left eye. It should be level with the patient's eye, and just far enough back to place his eye in shadow. Your own eye should be directly op-posite the patient's. You should learn to use your right eye to examine the patient's right eye, and your left one to examine his left. This will avoid nasal bumps. Try to hold your breath, especially during the direct examination. Having placed the patient, the light and yourself in position, proceed first with the indirect examination. With yourself about fifteen inches in front of the patient, place the ophthalmoscope in front of your eye, look through the sight-hole, direct the mirror towards the light, and then rotate it so as to re-flect the light into the eye to be examined. Have the patient look past your right ear if you are examining his right eye, and vice versa. This is for the purpose of bringing his optic disk into your line of vision. The optic disk should always be selected as the starting point of an ophthalmoscopic exam-ination; it being the least sensitive part of the fundus, throwing light from the mirror upon it will not cause the pupil to contract, nor is the patient alarmed by the bright light as he would be if you first directed the light upon the mac-ula lutea. Many changes due to disease manifest themselves in the disk. It is a very striking object in the fundus, and one soon learns to distinguish it clear-ly and notice slight changes from the normal. When the eye is illuminated, which fact will be manifested by the pupil changing from black to red, you should take the object lens between the index finger and thumb and place it before the patient's eye, rest your little finger on his forehead, holding the lens at about its focal length from his eye, and, while keeping the fundus il-luminated, move the lens to and from the eye, at the same time rotating it on its vertical axis sufficiently to throw the reflected images of the light out of your visual line. If by these movements a clear image of the optic disk is not formed, then move the lens up and down, or from side to side, until a sharp image of the disk is seen, apparently on and in the center of the lens. The im-age is not formed on the lens but at about its focal length in front of it. With this method we get a brightly illuminated large field, but the details of the fundus will be smaller than with the direct method. A little practice should make one expert in this method. For practice, it would be well at first to se-lect eyes with large pupils, and especially those that have been dilated by some mydriatic, homatropine being the best for this purpose, as the effects of a weak solution will pass off in two days. Cocaine will answer if the eye is young. The small pupil and the less transparent lens, which are generally found in the eyes of old persons, render them not so suitable for practice as are the eyes of younger persons. Examine all the eyes you can. Do this on account of the great variation of the normal fundus. By indirect ophthalmoscopy, the optic disk and retinal vessels appear larger in hyperopia than in emmetropia, and smaller in myopia.

The next point in the fundus to be examined is the macula lutea. Have the patient look straight forward, and direct your own eye slightly to one side of the center of the cornea to escape the reflection from its center, which would prevent you seeing the macula distinctly. A slight lateral movement of the lens will also help you to see this region. Around the macula you will notice a luminous silvery ring, though it varies greatly in shape, size and distinctness in different eyes, and will often change its form and size when it is being observed, owing to the play of light from the ophthalmoscope. In the center of this will be noticed a small, round spot or dot, called the fovea centralis. The color of the fovea varies, being sometimes quite dark and sometimes quite light. This halo, or reflex, is not seen in all eyes; it is best seen in young eyes, seldom or never in the eyes of the very old. After you have examined the macula have the patient direct his eye up and down, right and left, up and to the right, up and to the left, down and to the right, down and to the left; this will bring all parts of the fundus into view. Notice with care the condition of the vessels, their color, the sharpness of their edges, whether they are covered or displaced in any part of their course, their pulsation, their degree of torturosity and the " light streak." You must also observe with great care the condition of the macula and of the fovea, besides the general appearance of the fundus, its color and general regular contour, degree and variety of pigmentation, which varies greatly in different parts, and also notice the number and state of the choroidal vessels. The choroidal vessels can be easily distinguished from the retinal vessels. They are broader, less sharply defined, and look flat and ribbon-like. They lack the reflex streak, and they form, by their numerous anastomoses, a dense network with oblong meshes. Also notice the state of the vitreous humor, whether fluid or solid, and whether it contains any opacities; if so, note the extent and rate of their independent movements. Look, also, for any detachment of the retina which may exist. Do not neglect any of these points, but examine each eye carefully.

If you are presbyopic, or have any refractive defect that prevents you from seeing an object at twelve inches, you will have to correct it either by spectacles or by the correcting lenses found in the disk of the ophthalmoscope. A strong plus lens is sometimes placed behind the sight-hole of the ophthalmoscope for the purpose of magnifying the image of the fundus; but this is not advisable, for it is apt to dim the outlines of the image. It is better to use a weaker object lens, which gives a large image and a small field. A three-inch lens is the best for general purposes.

Direct ophthalmoscopy, while very simple, requires practice. In this method the mirror is used without the lens, the observer looking directly into the eye under observation. To this he places the mirror before his own eye, and tilts it so that it receives the rays of light from the lamp and reflects them into the patient's eye. The mirror should be brought as near as possible to the patient. The nearer we come to the pupil the larger will be the field of vision. We should try to place the mirror at the anterior focus of the patient's eye. Practise until you can do this, as it will save much calculation in testing refraction by this method. The principal difficulty the novice encounters is in relaxing the accommodation, being conscious that the object is very near. The art of relaxing the accommodation when looking at a near-by object can be gained by reading with each eye singly through a strong plus glass, say 4 D., held at its focal distance, which is 25 cm., taking care all the while that the other eye remains open, though covered by a screen. This, in case you are emmetropic; if not, render yourself so by the use of the proper glasses. If the patient is emmetropic, and the observer can relax his accommodation, he will see the fundus as soon as he illuminates it. By this method the fundus appears of a lighter color, the disk whiter, and the "light streak" of the vessels very bright and clear. Details of the fundus will be seen that were invisible by the indirect method. For detecting pathological changes and testing refraction this method of ophthalmoscopy is superior to any other. If you can not relax your accommodation, then you must place a minus lens behind the sight-hole of the ophthalmoscope. Make it sufficiently strong to enable you to clearly see the details of the fundus, weakening it from time to time until you can relax your accommodation. If the patient be myopic, you will have to use a minus lens to see his fundus. If hyperopic, you should use a plus lens; although you could make use of your power of accommodation, it would not be well to do so. It might interfere with your forming the habit of seeing with relaxed accommodation. By this method the macula lutea will have no halo, but there will appear, in some cases, a small horseshoe-shaped reflection from the fovea centralis, which will appear very much larger than by the indirect examination. Your position, as well as that of the patient and of the light, should be the same as in the indirect method, except you should be much nearer the patient, and for this reason you should sit with your legs turned to one side of the patient, changing from one side to the other as you change from one eye to the other. The parts of the fundus should be examined in the same order as indicated for the indirect method; but have the patient move his eye very slowly, because the field of view is very small, with the details highly magnified. The cornea, lens and vitreous should all be examined as you approach the eye when illuminating it. The slightest changes of structure are discovered by this method.

Chapter Ten - The Diagnosis and Correction of Anomalies of Refraction and Accommodation

Preliminary to the consideration of the anomalies of refraction and accommodation, a brief consideration of the emmetropic eye and the function of accommodation and convergence will be of value. The normally refracting, or emmetropic, eye is one whose principal focus coincides with its retina. It is adapted to parallel rays of light, and when its accommodation is at rest its refractive power will bring such rays to a focus on its retina, all rays coming from a greater distance than five metres being considered as parallel. Such an eye will see all objects at and beyond this distance distinctly, provided the acuity of vision is normal, that the objects subtend to an angle of five minutes, and that they are sufficiently illuminated and contrasted and continue before the eye a sufficient length of time to influence the retina. The emmetropic eye is the ideal eye, both in its structure and in its functions, and it is the standard by which the anomalies of refraction must be estimated. No other refraction of the eye is capable of giving to the region of accommodation so great an extent. In a strictly mathematical sense, emmetropia, in all probability, does not exist. The refractive surfaces of the different meridians of the cornea, or lens, are seldom or never the same, and slight degrees of myopia do not manifest themselves during an ordinary examination. In youth, slight degrees of hypermetropia are hard to prove, and even if the eye be emmetropic, with the accommodation paralyzed, it may be myopic when the muscle of accommodation resumes its normal tone. In practice, we are justified in considering all eyes emmetropic when the error does not exceed one-fifth of a dioptre. In order to see distinctly an object situated nearer than infinity, it is necessary for the emmetropic eye to increase its refractive power; this power or function is called accommodation. It is a product of muscular energy, and varies with the age and health of the individual. We cannot draw a sharp line between it and its anomalies. The terms range of accommodation, amplitude of accommodation and force of accommodation are used synonymously by different writers, and must be clearly differentiated from the term region of accommodation. The first three terms — range, amplitude and force of accommodation — mean its power. The dioptric power of a lens, the focal length of which coincides with the near point ot an emmetropic eye, measures and expresses its range, amplitude or power of accommodation. The second term — region of accommodation — means the space in which accommodation is exercised, and it represents the distance between the near and far point of distinct vision. Along a certain part of the visual line different objects seem to be seen with a given amount of accommodation. This part is called the line of accommodation, and its length varies; if the eye is accommodated for its near point it will be very short. The external ocular muscles have the power of directing the visual lines to a point, thus enabling one to see an object singly and at the same time with both eyes. This power is termed convergence, and is intimately related to accommodation. As a rule, when emmetropic eyes are directed to a given point, they are accommodated for that point. Yet, bear in mind, this relationship is not absolute, but variable. The range of accommodation is divided into absolute, binocular and relative. The absolute represents the greatest power of accommodation that can be exercised by one eye alone. The binocular range is the range with both eyes converged to one point, and that the nearest point of distinct and single vision. The relative range is the range over which we have control at a given convergence of the visual lines; it represents the degree in which accommodation is dependent on convergence. Its amount may be measured by prisms which vary the convergence while the eye is accommodated for a given distance, or by lenses which change the range of accommodation with the visual axis converging to a given point. The positive-relative range of accommodation represents the power of accommodation that can be exercised at a distance nearer than the point of convergence. The relative range is of importance, from the fact that the accommodation can be maintained only for a distance at which, in reference to the negative, the positive part of the relative range is tolerably great.

Tension of accommodation is the normal or physiological contraction of the ciliary muscle. Spasm of accommodation is an abnormal contraction of the ciliary muscle; it may be tonic or clonic. Binocular vision is a function that should be studied at some length, on account of its complexity and importance and the amount of reflex trouble and consequent suffering which any disturbance of this function may cause. Physiology teaches that a line drawn from an object through the nodal point to the fovea centralis is called the visual line, that the fovea is the most highly developed part of the retina for "form sense," and that an object situated at the intersection of the visual lines, and having its images formed in the fovea centralis of both eyes, will appear as a single object. The corresponding parts of the two retinae have their identical points where two ocular images appear as one.

Binocular vision offers the following advantages:

(1) The field of vision is considerably larger than that of one eye.

(2) The perception of depth is rendered easier, as the retinal images are obtained from two different points.

(3) A more perfect estimate of the distance and size of an object can be formed in consequence of the perception of the degree of convergence.

To have and maintain perfect and comfortable binocular vision, the visual axis must be easily directed to and kept at one point; the magnitude of the retinal images should be the same, of equal distinctness and of the same color. If the variation and distinctness of the ocular images is great, it may render binocular vision poorer than monocular. The double ocular impression must be conveyed to the brain, then by a psychical act be projected into space, and at the intersection of the visual lines caused to unite and form a single erect image corresponding to the form and position of the object in space. The structures and functions that take part in the binocular vision are many, including the refractive and muscular systems of the eye, the retina, the optic nerve, the brain, the cellular tissues of the orbit, the capsule of Tenon, the conjunctiva and numerous reflex functions. The stimulus of binocular vision is evidently due to the retinal images being received on corresponding or near-by points of the two retinae, and an associated movement of the eyes, which appears to be an inherited function that varies with the individual and is increased by practice. When the deviation of the visual lines is great, the ocular images are formed at widely separated points of the two retinae, and, as a consequence, there is a great difference in the nervous impressions produced by them, and there is very little tendency to fuse them. The more widely the images are separated the less suffering and confusion they cause, and there is a marked tendency for the eyes to deviate still more, thus causing one of the images to be formed on a more slightly sensitive part of the retina, enabling it to be unnoticed and forgotten. When this takes place binocular vision ceases to exist, the patient, being relieved of the pain and suffering caused by trying to maintain binocular vision, accepts monocular vision with the belief that his eyesight has improved. Eyes which differ from the emmetropic eye in their refractive powers are, as already stated, called ametropic. Of ametropia there are two main divisions, hyperopia and myopia. Hypermetropic eyes will bring converging rays of light to a focus upon their retinae with relaxed accommodation. Under the same conditions, myopic eyes will bring diverging rays of light to a focus upon their retinae. An eye whose refractive media differs in power in its several sections or meridians is termed astigmatic. Refractive errors are classified into manifest and latent, false and true, depending upon the state of the ciliary muscle, which sometimes keeps in a persistent state of contraction even when the visual line is directed to infinity. To know that the accommodation is at rest, it is generally necessary to paralyze the ciliary muscle. The drugs that have the power of doing this are called mydriatics.

The various refractive errors are divided as follows:

Hyperopia into Congenital and Acquired; Manifest, Latent and Total; Faculative, Relative and Absolute; Axial, Index, Curvature.

Myopia into Congenital and Acquired; Progressive and Stationary; Manifest, False and True; Axial, Index, Curvature.

Astigmatism into Congenital and Acquired; Manifest, False and True; Corneal and Lenticular; Regular and Irregular. The regular is divided into simple hyperopic and simple myopic, and mixed astigmatism. The measurements of the various refractive and accommodative conditions are determined by Dioptrometry.

Dioptrometry is divided into subjective and objective methods. In the subjective method we consider the rays of light that radiate from some external object and form an image on the patient's retina.

Except for the power we have of changing the direction of these rays, by changing the distance of the test object or by interposing a lens, we must depend upon the answers of the patient for our data. And his answers will depend upon his power of perception, interpretation and expression, assuming that he is truthful and does not wish to deceive us. To derive accurate knowledge from this method of dioptrometry, we need test objects of known size and form, placed at a definite distance, and arranged in such a way that their form must be distinguished before they can be named. This method is based upon the visual acuity, and in determining the refraction we also determine the acuteness of vision. The first step in this examination is to determine the far point of distinct vision, and by that means to find the kind of rays for which the eye is adapted. In spite of its drawbacks this method is of greatest clinical value. No matter what other method we may use to determine the refraction of the eye, the subjective method, with the test object placed at a distance of at least five meters, must always be used before prescribing glasses. To make use of this method, we require, in addition to a series of test objects, a case of convex and concave spherical and cylindrical

TEST-TYPES.

D-050

LEFT	COOT	FELT	FOOD
COOL	FEET	CLOD	LOLL
FEEL	LODE	DEFT	SOTO
DOLL	YELL	TOOL	CELT

D-075

COO	LEE	OLD	ELF
FEE	COD	LET	TOD
ODD	EEL	TOO	OFF
ELL	DOT	FOE	COT

D-100

LEET	COLT	LOFT
FOLD	FEED	DELL
TOLL	TOLD	FOOL
DOLE	FELL	FLOE

D-150

CODE	DOLT
FLED	LOOT
COLD	DOLL

D-200

FED	LOO
ODE	TOE
LOT	OFT

lenses, with trial frames to hold them and a stenopaic slit and hole. The test objects that have been found to be of the greatest value are a series of letters, figures, dots and lines, arranged in such a manner and of such a form and size that when placed at the distance indicated by their number, in either metres or feet, each separate part of the object will form an angle on the examined retina of one minute, the various parts of the test object being separated by this distance. A single dot, or square, or line subtending to such an angle would not serve as a test. There must be at least two dots, and they must be separated by a distance equal to their breadth, neither more nor less. Numerous investigators have shown that, in order to recognize objects as forms, the average normal human eye requires that they be of such a size and placed at such a distance from the eye as to subtend to an angle of one minute; the distance between two test objects should also form this angle. This applies to black objects on a white ground. On this data Snelling based his test types. They are composed of black letters (on a white ground) of such a size that the whole letter will form an angle of five minutes and each separate limb of each letter will form an angle of one minute, when hung at the distance indicated by their number. They are numbered from .25 of a metre to 60 metres. To measure the acuity of vision, and find the far point, place the type at the distance indicated by its number and have the patient read it. If he reads the indicated type at his far point his acuity of vision is normal. It is quite important that the letters be arranged in an irregular manner, so that they do not form words, and that the paper and type should present a rough, dead surface. This is of great importance in the smaller types that are used to test accommodation, the regular reflection from a polished surface being very annoying; nor do the rays from such a surface correspond in divergence

D.=V.

E O F C T D L

D.=VII₁₁.

C T O E D F

D.=X.

F D E C L

D.=XV.

O L C F

with the distance at which the type is held. On account of the irregularities in Snelling's scale, several others have constructed series of test types, the most prominent being Monyer's and Green's. Aside from the more regular interval, these types have no advantage over those of Snelling, and as any test type can give us only the average visual acuity, and as Snelling's types are in general use and well-made, and when there is a necessity of variation in the scale of Snelling's type it can be made by changing their distance from the eye, they are on the whole the best for practical work. Another test type, called Jaeger's, was much in use in former times and are still used by some oculists in testing near vision, but they are not constructed or arranged in a scientific manner and no accurate measurements can be made with them; they are useful when, after correction, we wish to ascertain if the glasses are comfortable by having the patient read for some little time, yet even for this purpose a newspaper would be a more practical test. Snelling's other tests, the dots, figures and lines, constructed on the same principle as his letters, are used to test children's eyes and the eyes of such persons as cannot read. For determining astigmatism, radiating and parallel lines are used; these are constructed on the same principle as the test letters, although the divisions of the scale are not so fine. The trial lenses that are used for this method of dioptometry are numbered to correspond with spectacle glasses. Lenses used for spectacles are, at the present day, numbered according to the new or metric system. This has for its unit a lens of one metre focal length, and of a refractive power of one dioptre; this is expressed by the sign D. In this system the refractive power of the lens is expressed, not its focal length. When we wish to find the focal length, we have but to remember that 2 D., being twice as strong as 1 D., its focal length will be half as long as the unit, or one-half a metre; 10 D., being ten times as strong as 1 D., the focal length of such a lens would be one-tenth of a metre. Where it is required to translate from the old inch system to the metric system we consider 40 English inches equal to one metre, and, to obtain the dioptric strength, we divide forty by the number of the lens in inches. For instance, if the lens were

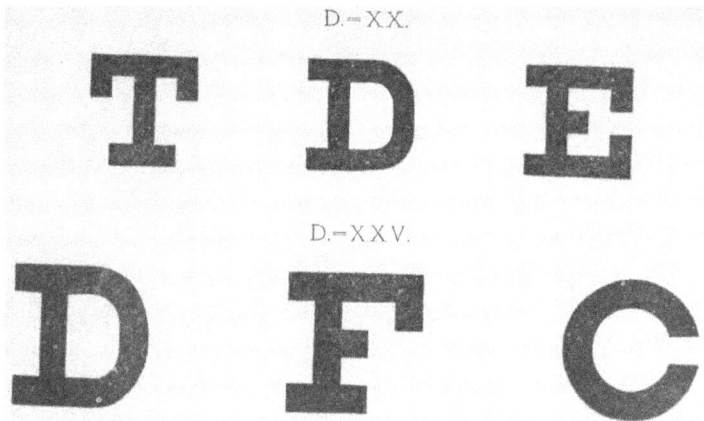

D.—XX.

T D E

D.—XXV.

D F C

one of one tenth, or ten inches focal length, we divide forty by ten, which gives four as being the dioptric strength of the lens. The old system had so many faults it has justly fallen into disuse. A complete case of trial glasses should contain forty-five pairs of convex and concave cylindrical glasses. The weaker lenses, up to 7 D., should be separated by an interval not greater than .25 D. The weakest lens should be .12 D. and the strongest .25 D. in the sphericals, while in the cylindrical the series should be. 25 D. to 10 D. The frame to hold these lenses should be adjustable to the height of the nose and the width of the face, and also be capable of bringing the centers of the glasses opposite the center of the eyes. In addition, it should be graduated in degrees, so as to define the position of the axis of the cylindrical lenses, and it should be as light as possible. In addition, the case should contain three disks of metal, one to serve as a screen for the eye under examination, one with a stenopaic slit 1.5 mm. in width, and one with a stenopaic hole 1.5 mm. in diameter. The disks should be the size of the test lenses, so as to fit into the same frame, and they should be of a dull black. A card of Snelling's test-types, graded from four to sixty metres, is the kind that is used to test refraction, together with a small card, graded from .25 to 3 metres, for testing the near point. This includes all the apparatus necessary for this method of subjective dioptometry. To determine the refraction, we hang the test-card in a position where it will be illuminated by diffuse daylight — never by the direct rays of the sun. If daylight is not available, use artificial light, taking care that it is properly diff used and that it is of an amount equal to diffuse daylight, because the test-types are adapted to that kind of light. The patient should be placed at a distance of at least five metres from the card, with his face turned away from the light; nor should the light be allowed to fall on the back of his trial spectacles, as that would cause an annoying reflection that would often blur the vision. At whatever distance the patient is placed, it should correspond to the number of the line of type that is to be read as the standard of measurement. If number five is to be used, he should be five metres from the card; if number six is used he should be six metres from the card, and so on, but never less than five metres. He should be seated on a comfortable, firm chair, and the height of the standard line of type should be the same as that of his eyes, and surface of the card should be parallel with the plane of his face. The trial case should be on a table within easy reach. The glasses should be kept clean,

D.=XXX.

D.=XXXV.

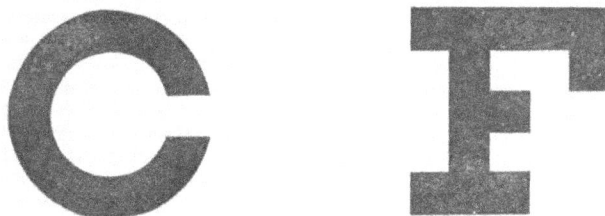

D.=XL.

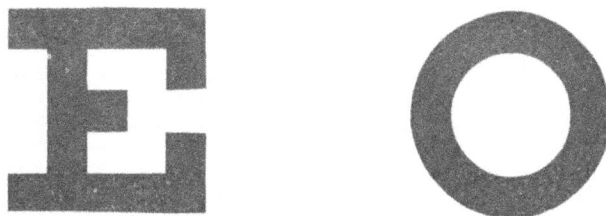

as a slight film of dirt will impair the sight and may be the cause of error. Allow the patient to become used to the illumination of the room in which the examination is to be made, and, if he has been subject to an ophthalmoscopic examination, wait at least fifteen minutes before attempting to test his refraction. If he is suffering from an acute inflammation of the eye, postpone the test, if possible, until you have relieved the acute symptoms. Each eye should be tested separately, and the eye that is not in use should be covered by an opaque screen, taking care that no pressure is made on the eyeball, as that would impair the vision for a time. See that the eye which is being examined is opened. Nipping the lids will often impair the test. To do rapid and accurate work, it is requisite to have a systematic and habitual manner of testing. Cover the patient's left eye and have him direct the right eye to the test-card, which, we assume, has been placed five metres distant. Have him read the letters on the card, beginning with the largest line of type. Make a note of the smallest line he can read. This line will indicate the acuity of vision for his right eye. Make the same test of his left eye, and then with both eyes together, and note the result. If he reads the test-type number five at five metres, he has the average normal acuity of vision. In recording the results, take the distance at which the smallest line of letters is seen as the numerator of a fraction, and the number of the line that is read at this distance as the denominator. For instance, if number five has been read at five metres by the right eye, write that the vision of the right is 5/5 — *i.e.*, normal. If number ten was read at this distance, the vision would be 5/10, or one-half the normal. Do not reduce the fraction, because it indicates the distance at which the test was made, and this knowledge is of great importance in estimating possible errors due to convergence and accommodation. The next step in the examination is to find whether plus or minus spherical glasses improve vision, and whether the stenopaic slit or hole improves it or makes it worse, turning the slit about in various directions and noting the results. You will also note whether the patient sees some letters better than others, both being of the same size. Then take the test-card, which is arranged as a clock dial, with a series of parallel lines — generally three in number — running in various directions, from one to twelve, corresponding with the divisions of the clock face — note whether he sees any one of these groups of lines more distinctly than others.

If so, try to make all the lines equally distinct to him by the use of cylindrical lenses, and note whether, at the same time, they improve his vision for the test-types. If vision is improved, or not made worse, by lenses or the stenopaic slit or hole, we assume that the patient has a manifest refractive defect. If plus spherical glasses improve, or do not make vision worse at a distance, it is a case of manifest hyperopia. If minus spherical glasses improve vision at a distance, it is a case of manifest myopia, either false or true. If cylinders or the stenopaic slit or hole improve vision, it is a case of manifest astigmatism, either false or true. All of this we will consider in detail under the treatment of the various refractive errors. In recording these tests of vision, writers use the sign O. D. to denote the right eye, and the sign O. S. to denote the left eye, and the sign O. U. to denote both eyes together. The following will serve as an example of a report of an examination of the visual acuity and refraction:

O. D. $\frac{5}{6}$? ? $+$ I D. $\frac{5}{6}$? O. U. $\frac{5}{6}$

the question marks indicating the number of letters in a given line that were

O. S. $\frac{5}{10}$ $+$ 2 D. $\frac{5}{6}$

not read correctly. The translation would be as follows: The right eye, with a plus lens of one dioptre, read the line of test-type marked 5 metres at a distance of 5 metres, failing on one letter of that line. The left eye, with a plus lens of two dioptres, read the line marked 6 metres at a distance of 5 metres. You will notice in this example that vision is not normal before or after correction with either eye alone, but that with (O. U.) both eyes together there is the normal amount of vision. This is frequently the case. On the other hand, sometimes the vision of the eyes combined is poorer than either eye singly. In such cases some lack of muscular balance is apt to exist. To measure the accommodation, we find the nearest point at which the patient can read, distinctly, type of such a size that it would subtend to an angle of five minutes when held at eight Paris inches or twenty centimetres from the eye. Remember, this is only a clinical or practical test, but it is of great value in prescribing glasses for near vision. The distance of eight inches was selected by Donders as the distance at which fine type should be read. Having found the distance for each eye, separately indicate it by the capital P. (punctum proximum). P. indicates the distance at which it was read either in centimetres or inches. An example:

O. D. P. = 22 c. c.
O. S. P. = 8 in.
O. U. P. = 25 c. c.

The location of the far point by the test-type alone, when it is less than five metres, is too often neglected. The knowledge of the position of this point will often save time in finding the correct glass, and will serve as a check, and may prevent one's mistaking false for true myopia.

Chapter Eleven - Objective Dioptometry

The Determination of Refraction by the Ophthalmoscope.

The principal instrument used in objective dioptometry is the ophthalmoscope. The determination of the refractive conditions of the eye by this instrument is termed ophthalmoscopic dioptometry, or dioptoscopy. There are three methods of dioptoscopy. These are termed direct ophthalmoscopy, skiascopy and indirect ophthalmoscopy. There are certain advantages in objective dioptometry. The primary one is its ability to show the refractive condition of the eye examined, independent of the statements of the patient or the amount of vision of the eye. Second, in measuring the amount of elevation or depression of a given part of the fundus. Third, in distinguishing spasm from myopia. The ability to determine these several things varies with the method used and with the skill of the ophthalmologist. To offset these advantages there are several disadvantages to this method. First, the absolute inability to determine the normal tension of the accommodation. Second, the great difficulty of measuring the refraction at the fovea centralis. Third, the great uncertainty in measuring small errors of refraction. In prescribing glasses for the correction of errors of refraction, objective dioptrometry must never be used to the exclusion of the subjective method. Subject to the exceptions here mentioned, objective dioptrometry is of great value, not only in testing refraction, but also in measuring normal and pathological elevations and depressions in the fundus of the eye. Direct ophthalmoscopy and skiascopy are of most value, and next in importance come indirect ophthalmoscopy and ophthalmometry. We will first consider skiascopy, or the fundus reflex test, because it requires less study and less practice than direct ophthalmoscopy. Its synonyms are feratoscopy, retinoscopy, koroscopy, urnbrascopy, shadow test, etc., skiascopy, or the fundus reflex test, being the best names. Bowman (1859) was the first to use this method. He used it for the detection of conical cornea. In a communication to Donders (1864) he mentioned having used it in detecting astigmatism. After that it seems to have fallen into disuse. Cuignet (1873) revived it, but he was not able to explain the optical principles governing it, so it remained for a long time without general recognition of its value. In skiascopy there are two methods: In one a plane mirror is used, and in the other a concave mirror, the plane mirror method being the more exact of the two methods — though not the one in general use — we will describe it first.

The room in which the examination is made should be dark, in the sense that no light is to be admitted except that used for the examination, and that may be a lamp, gas or electric light, the first two mentioned being preferred on account of their larger surface of flame. The best position for the observer will be five metres from the patient, as the patient will not be so apt to accommodate unduly at this distance. The light is best placed a few inches from the mirror and shaded so that the patient's eyes will receive only rays from the mirror, which should be 'held before the observer's eye; this mirror being a plane ophthalmoscopic mirror, having a sight-hole of about 3 mm. The mirror should be turned so as to receive the light and reflect the rays into the patient's eye, causing the eye to glow. By noting the direction, extent and rapidity of movement, the sharpness of the shadow's outline and the distinctness of the ocular luster, we determine the kind and, to a certain extent, the amount of refractive error. In emmetropia, the luster and the shadow move in the same direction that the mirror is rotated, the movement being rapid and of great extent, the glow bright and the outlines of the shadow distinct. In hyperopia, the shadow also moves with the mirror. The greater the amount of hyperopia the less distinct is the shadow. The extent and rate of movement of the shadows decrease as the hyperopia increases. In myopia the shadow moves in the opposite direction to the movement of the mirror; and, as in hyperopia, the greater the error the less will be the movement and distinctness of the shadow's outline. In simple and compound hyperopic astigmatism, the movement of the shadow will be in the same direction as that of the mirror, but will differ in amount and extent in different meridians of rotation. If the principal meridians are vertical and horizontal, the shadow will move more rapidly in one of these meridians than in the other, but always in the same direction. If the principal meridians are oblique, the shadow will move obliquely across the path of rotation. In simple myopic astigmatism, the shadow will move in two directions, with the mirror in the emmetropic meridian and against the mirror in the myopic meridian. In compound myopic astigmatism, the shadow will move against the mirror in both meridians, but will differ in extent and rapidity. The movements of the shadow in mixed astigmatism resemble those of myopic astigmatism, but the extent and rate of movement in the two opposite meridians are not so great. The shadow is never so clearly outlined in astigmatism as in the other refractive conditions. By the mirror alone we can establish the diagnosis of refractive errors and approximate their amount. To measure the amount of refractive error, a series of convex and concave lenses is required. These must be placed before the patient's eye, one at a time, and the weakest that reverses the shadow will indicate the amount of error. The kind of lenses to be used will depend upon the refractive condition. For hyperopia use plus lenses, for myopia use minus lenses. In astigmatism each meridian must be corrected separately. To discover the axis of the correcting glass in astigmatism, the axis of rotation of the mirror must coincide with the principal meridians of the cornea. This method of examination necessitates a room five metres long, but! it is the simplest and best, and more nearly approaches the subjective method than any of the others. In spasm of accommodation it must give precedence to direct ophthalmoscopy. The shadow test with the concave mirror is made as follows: The light is placed above the patient's head, while the observer, seated a little more than a metre from the patient, illuminates the eye, rotating the mirror from side to side and up and down. The movements of the shadow will be in the reverse direction from those in the plane mirror method. In emmetropia and hyperopia and myopia, of less than one dioptre, the movement of the shadow will be against that of the mirror. In myopia of one dioptre there will be no movement of the shadow, the eye seeming to light up from all sides and to grow dim in the same way.

Diagnoses of refractive errors are made by this method in the same way as by the plane mirror method, with the above-named exception. In this method a myopia of one dioptre is taken as a standard, and for this reason a plus one dioptre must be substracted from the glass which causes the movements of the shadow to reverse. If a plus two changes the movement, there is a hyperopia of one dioptre. If a minus two changes the movement, there is a myopia of three dioptres. If a plus one changes the movement, the refraction is emmetropic. The same principle holds good in astigmatism. The reason why the movements in the concave mirror methods are reversed, as compared with those of the plane mirror method, is that the plane mirror is itself the luminous object from which the retinal image is formed, the shadow of which we see moving across the pupillary space. With the concave mirror the inverted image of the lamp, which is formed at the focus of the mirror, becomes the object for the retinal image. The optical principles governing skiascopy are very simple. The plane mirror is held so as to reflect into the eye of the patient the rays of light it receives from the lamp. If the mirror is five metres from the patient's eye we call all the rays parallel, and if he is emmetropic they will be brought to a focus on his retina, forming there an inverted image of the lamp. Parallel rays emerge from his eye and are brought to a focus on the observer's retina, forming there an upright image. If the mirror be rotated to the left, the retinal image formed on the patient's fundus will move towards the right of the fundus.

The movement towards the patient's right (our left) will cause the image formed on our retina to move to its right side, and, following the law of mental projection, it will be projected towards, and seem to move, to our left. The same would hold good if the patient were hyperopia When he is myopic, rays of light issuing from his fundus are converging, and, consequently, they come to a focus in front of his eye. In this case we do not see the image formed on his fundus, but the aerial image of it, which is formed at his far point. This image is, of course, inverted, and will move in a reverse direction to the movement of the retinal image. This aerial image, being the observer's object, its mentally projected image will correspond in movement with it. The concave mirror method is not quite so simple. In it diverging rays of light are reflected by the mirror and changed into converging rays, which cross and form an image of the lamp beyond the focus of the mirror. When the mirror is rotated to the left, this image also moves to the observer's left (the patient's right). This image is the object for the patient, and its movement towards his right will cause it to form an image on the left side of his retina. Now, if the refraction of the eye is emmetropic, rays will issue from the left side of his fundus and form an image on the left side of the observer's retina, and this will be projected to and move towards the observer's right. In myopia we have simply to consider another inverted image; consequently the final movement will be towards the left, that is, in the same direction as the rotation of the mirror. Skiascopy is of great value in testing the eyes of children and of those who can not read. It is also of value as a check on other methods in testing the eyes of ignorant and stupid persons. In case of spasm of accommodation, it is necessary to paralyze the accommodation, and, while this enables one to measure the total refraction of the eye, the accompanying dilatation of the pupil is a disadvantage, inasmuch as it brings the peripheral portions of the refracting media into action. These peripheral portions are generally of greater refractive power than the more central portions. In some cases there exists a marked difference; especially is this true of astigmatic cases. A dilated pupil is also apt to bring into play a certain amount of spherical aberration and irregular astigmatism. Probably the greatest advantage skiascopy has over direct ophthalmoscopy is that the observer does not have to relax his accommodation. Ability to measure the refractive condition of the eye by means of direct ophthalmoscopy should be acquired, even if one never intends to use this method in estimating ametropia. It is by the direct methods that tumors, exudations or excavations of the fundus are measured and their rate of growth noted. By no other method can this be done.

To perfect one's self in the use of direct ophthalmoscopy requires time, thought and practice, although there are no real difficulties to be overcome unless one makes them for himself by struggling to relax his accommodation. The first essential in this method is for the observer to know the refraction of his own eye, and if error exists to correct it. Hyperopia and myopia can be corrected by the lenses found in the disk of the ophthalmoscope. For the correction of astigmatism a special lens, mounted in a clip, can be swung in front of the lens disk, or one may wear spectacles to correct the defect, the extra lens being the best device, as it allows the ophthalmoscope to be brought nearer the observer's eye. The patient selected for practice should be one whose refractive media are clear. His pupil should be dilated and his accommodation paralyzed, so that the observer will have no reason to think that the patient is using his accommodation. The observer should place the ophthalmoscope before his eye and look into the patient's eye, bringing the mirror as close as possible to the patient's eye, at the same time keeping it well illuminated. The best part of the fundus to select for the purpose of examination is the temporal edge of the optic disk. If the observer's accommodation is at rest (the patient being emmetropic), he should see the edge of the disk clearly and sharply defined, every little irregularity standing out bold and distinct. Merely seeing the details of the fundus is not sufficient; they must be seen with great vividness. If the observer does not see them in this way he should not make any effort to see more clearly, for if he does he will accommodate and so defeat his object. He must simply allow both eyes to open and look passively at the dark wall with his unoccupied eye. If this does not produce a distinct image, he may know that he is using his accommodation, and he must then place a minus glass in front of the sight-hole, starting with the weakest and rotating stronger and stronger ones before his eye until he sees distinctly. Having sharply denned the disk's edge, he should view the other parts of the fundus, changing the lens as the elevations of the fundus vary. Having convinced himself that he can clearly distinguish the details of the fundus, he should begin at the edge of the disk, trying a weaker lens than before, and so continue using a weaker and weaker lens until he can make the examination without the use of one. He will find that in this way he will soon get control of his accommodation. He should not take hyperopic or astigmatic cases, nor a case with a small pupil, for his first examinations. Having become expert in seeing the fundus by the direct method, he should endeavor to measure the refraction along the visual line. To do this, it is necessary to take some other portion of the fundus than the fovea centralis, it being a poor object, on account of its having no markings or distinct outline to focus. The surrounding macula is also a poor object on account of the great thickness of the retina encircling it. At this portion of the fundus the retina is about five-tenths of a millimetre in thickness, while at the fovea (the center of distinct vision) it is only about two-tenths of a millimetre in thickness. The best object to select is a small retinal vessel, one that gives off branches about two millimetres from the macula lutea. The retina at this point being about three-tenths of a millimetre in thickness, and the vessel dipping somewhat below its level, the increased thickness of the choroid at this point makes the difference between its level and the level of the fovea very slight. Even if the difference in level equalled one-twentieth of a millimetre, the difference in the amount of refraction would only equal one-sixth of a dioptre. To determine if this vessel is focused, the examiner must observe the light streak, noting if it stands out clear and bright, as it will when the vessel is sharply focused. The lens that enables one to see this clearly will practically define the condition of the refraction of the eye. If seen best without a lens, both the observer's and patient's accommodation being at rest, then the eye is emmetropic. To determine the exact amount of ametropia in a given case: If a plus lens is used, subtract from its focal length the distance of the lens from the principal point of the eye.

The same rule holds good in astigmatism. Where a vessel divides one can generally find branches which run at about right angles. The examiner should select this part and focus each branch. The difference in refraction of the branches will give the amount of astigmatism. This method is not so exact for astigmatism as for simple ametropia. It is of great value in detecting spasm of accommodation. Great authorities like Mauthner believe that spasm of the ciliary muscle always relaxes during a direct ophthalmoscopic examination. The enlargement of the image when the fundus is examined by the direct method is of great interest, the patient's eye acting as a simple microscope. In case the observer and the patient are both emmetropic, any object in the patient's fundus — the optic disk, for instance — will form an image on the observer's retina of the same size as the object irrespective of the distance separating their two eyes. The emmetropic observer would view the patient's optic disk under a visual angle of 5.7°. If the observer could distinctly see an object the diameter of the disk (1.5 mm.) held at 15 mm. from his principal point, it would appear under this visual angle. In other words, the patient's eye acts as a microscope of 15 mm. focal length. If the patient were hyperopia the enlargement would not be so great when viewed through the correcting lens of the ophthalmoscope. In myopia, under like conditions, it would appear larger. A distance of 250 mm. (or ten inches) has been assumed by American and English microscopists as the distance at which an object should be viewed to compare its retinal image with that of the retinal image formed by a magnifying instrument. If this comparison is used the image in direct ophthalmoscopy would be magnified 16 diameters. That is, the optic disk would seem 16 times as large as it would if it were viewed at ten inches from the observer's eye, without the use of the patient's dioptric media to magnify it. To find the number of times the optic disk, in emmetropia, is magnified by direct ophthalmoscopy, divide 250 mm. (the distance assumed for comparison) by 15 mm., the distance (in round figures) of the nodal point from the retina. The art of testing refraction by ophthalmoscopy having been acquired, elevations and depressions of the fundus can be easily determined. Every elevation will shorten the axis of the eye, while every depression will lengthen it. Shortening the axis of an emmetropic eye will cause it to become hyperopic, and vice versa. To determine the amount of lengthening or shortening, a normal part of the fundus should be examined, and preferably a part near the abnormal portion. Having found the refraction of this part of the fundus, the abnormal portion is to be measured, and the difference in the correcting glasses used will measure the amount of deviation of the abnormal from the normal part. To find the amount of shortening or lengthening of the eye, multiply the posterior focal length (expressed in millimetres) of the emmetropic eye by the anterior focal length (expressed in millimetres) and divide product by the focal length of the correcting glass (also expressed in millimetres); the quotient will indicate the increase of length in myopia and the decrease of length in hyperopia, if the correcting lens has been placed at the anterior principal point. Taking the values of the "reduced eye" for our data, posterior focal length, 20 mm., anterior focal length, 15 mm., we divide the product by the focal length of the correcting glass. For example: 20 multiplied by 15 equals 300; 300 divided by 1,000 equals three-tenths. Therefore three-tenths of a millimetre is the difference in length between a hyperopic or a myopic eye of one dioptre and an emmetropic eye. Three-tenths millimetres represents the amount of shortening in hyperopia and the amount of lengthening in myopia. It must be remembered that this gives the true measure only when the correcting lens is placed at the anterior principal point. If the lens is held at twenty-five millimetres from the principal point of the eye, which is about as near as it is possible to place it with the ordinary ophthalmoscope, this number, 25 mm., must be subtracted from the focal length of the correcting glass, if it be a convex lens, and added to its focal length, if it be a concave lens.

The following example will explain: Take 100 mm. as the focal length of the correcting lens, held at 25 mm. from the principal point. In hyperopia it would be worked out as follows:

$$\begin{array}{r} 100 \\ 25 \\ \hline 75)\overline{300} \\ \hline .4 \; 111111. \end{array}$$

95

Four millimetres being the amount of shortening of
the axis of the eye in a case of hyperopia equalling ten
dioptres, the lens being "held at twenty five millimetres from the principal point of the eye. In myopia the
distance is added, for example:

$$\begin{array}{r} 100 \\ 25 \\ \hline 125)\overline{300} \\ \hline \end{array}$$

$$2.4 \text{ mm.}$$

Two and four-tenths millimetres represent the
lengthening in such an eye. It is allowable to say, in a
general way, that three dioptres of refraction equal
one millimetre of shortening or lengthening of the eye. On account of the
great errors of refraction, caused by a slight difference in length of the optic
axis, direct ophthalmoscopy is a very sensitive and accurate way of measuring tumors, exudations, detachments, depressions or protrusions of the fundus of the eye. There are many other instruments used in objective dioptometry, but their importance to the general physician is not such as would warrant our giving a detailed description of them.

Clinical Consideration and Treatment of Ametropia
Hyperopia.

The hyperopic eye labors under the great disadvantage of being adapted
to the kind of rays of light which are seldom found in nature. Objects at a
great distance give off parallel rays, while objects near-by give off diverging
rays. For this reason the hyperopic eye is said to be suited to rays that come
from beyond infinity. Rays of this kind are the only ones the hyperopic eye is
capable of bringing to a focus on its retina, when its muscle of accommodation is at rest. As a consequence, the hyperope is forced to use his ciliary
muscle whenever he sees any object in this world distinctly. The nearer the
object, the greater the amount of accommodation necessary to see it. This
constant muscular strain sometimes gives rise to headaches and other dis-
tressing reflex nervous symptoms that are so promptly and brilliantly relieved by the use of glasses which neutralize the defect. The eyes of nearly all
young children are hyperopic. The sclerotic, which gives shape and support
to the eyeball, is very soft and tender in the young. For this reason young
children should never be required to read poor type, or do any fine work that
must be brought close to the eye. There are certain features of kindergarten
work that should be discouraged for this reason. Schoolrooms should be
brightly illuminated, as nothing is so harmful to children's eyes as being
forced to work in a poorly lighted room. The diagnosis of hyperopia is simple
and certain when the ciliary muscle is at rest. It is established when the patient sees objects situated at a distance as well or better through a convex
lens than without it. But the ciliary muscle is seldom at rest during life, and
its contraction may conceal a part or the whole of the defect. The portion that
can be detected by the subjective examination is termed manifest hyperopia;
that which remains concealed is termed latent hyperopia — the sum of the

manifest and the latent being termed total hyperopia. Sometimes the ciliary muscle is in such a state of spasmodic contraction that it not only hides all the hyperopia, but causes the eye to appear myopic. This condition is called pseudo-myopia. It may be detected by the ophthalmoscope, or with more certainty by paralyzing the ciliary muscle by Hydrobromate of Hyoscine. The terms facultative, relative and absolute hyperopia have reference to the amount of accommodation the patient can use to correct his hyperopia by means of his ciliary muscle and still have binocular vision. In relative hyperopia he can correct the defect by accommodation and undue convergence — in other words, he gives up binocular vision and squints in order to see objects distinctly. The absolute hyperope can not correct his hyperopia by any exercise of his power of accommodation or convergence. He can not see distinctly at any distance without convex glasses. The commonest form of hyperopia is the axial. In this form the eye is shorter in its antero-posterior diameter than an emmetropic eye whose refractive surface has the same curvature. In its higher degree it is often an undeveloped eye, being smaller in all its diameters. Index and curvature hyperopia are generally due to senile and pathological changes, aphakia, or absence of the crystalline lens, being a very common cause. Glaucoma is also one of the causes of acquired hyperopia. Many persons whose eyes are highly hyperopic seem to experience no trouble in using them. They may continue in this favorable state until age or an attack of illness compels them to resort to convex glasses in order to see distinctly. Others suffering from very slight, as well as those suffering from great, degrees of hyperopia seem to experience the greatest agony. Between these two extremes, patients present various degrees of annoyance and suffering. Some complain of blurring of vision after reading a short time. Others complain of headache after using the eyes or in the early morning; such patients may experience no blurring of the type when reading. A third class will have an attack of conjunctivitis, or blepharitis, every time they use their eyes for any length of time. In still another class of patients the symptoms are referred to parts of the body away from the eyes. The symptoms are all classed under the head of asthenopia. Strabismus convergens is often due to hyperopia, and is generally found in cases of moderate degree, and can often be cured by the wearing of glasses which correct the hyperopia. The determination of the form and amount of hyperopia requires careful testing and close attention to detail. In examination, both the subjective and objective methods should be used. First the subjective. Look at the patient's face; it will often appear flat, with the bridge of the nose poorly developed. The eyeballs may also appear small and flattened, and more freely movable than is the case with an emmetropic eye. Note if there is any tendency to squint. Have the patient relate his symptoms; question him as to the kind of work he does, and the amount. Also find out his idea as regards wearing spectacles. This last is of considerable importance, as some patients are eager to wear glasses while others are greatly averse to doing so. A simple statement to the first-named that it will be necessary for him to wear glasses would suffice. While in the case of the second patient, the reason why he should wear glasses and the danger following their non-use would have to be made clear to him or else he would be very apt to throw away your prescription and consult some quack, who would promise to cure him without spectacles. Then place your patient at five metres from the test-card of letters and record the vision of each eye separately. Then place convex glasses before the eye under examination. The strongest of the glasses with which he can see best gives the measure of the manifest hyperopia for that eye. Having found the manifest hyperopia for each eye separately, try them together, and note if the error is the same. Before concluding the examination have him read at his near point with these glasses with both eyes open, and notice whether he has comfortable binocular vision, and in how great a region he can read ordinary newspaper print. In pseudo-myopia, while the patient appears myopic he is hyperopic, and, when he is examined subjectively, he will reject all plus lenses, saying they make his vision worse, and will pick out minus ones, and see better with them at a distance: but, unlike a true myope, his far point and the focal length of the correcting glass will seldom coincide. The diagnosis can often be established by objective dioptrometry, as already explained. If you have any doubt, after the subjective and objective examinations, as to the kind or degree of error, then paralyze his accommodation. The best agent for this purpose is, in my opinion, Hydrobromate of Hyoscine, in solution of one to one hundred. Place one drop of this solution in the outer corner of each eye, direct the patient to close his eyes and remain quiet for half an hour; then he will be ready for the examination. An examination made at this time will reveal the total amount of hyperopia. The pupil being widely dilated, a disk with a hole about the diameter of his normal pupil should be placed before the eye while testing vision and refraction subjectively. Having by these several examinations determined the amount of manifest and latent hyperopia, you have next to consider the kind and strength of glasses, if any, that are to be prescribed, and when and how long they are to be worn. A great may things will have to be considered in this decision; for example, if he squints, if his power of accommodation is poor, if symptoms of asthenopia are marked, if his general health is poor, if he is compelled to use his eyes a great deal for near work, or if his vision is poor without glasses and good with them. Should he be a sufferer from spasm of accommodation, it will generally be necessary for him to wear glasses at all times, except when asleep. If the glasses do not make distant vision better, and the eyes and head simply grow tired or the type becomes dim, then glasses for near vision only need be used. Persons who spend a great deal of time out of doors are better off without glasses for distant vision, unless it is greatly improved by them. This is emphatically true if they live in a crowded city and have to go about at night. Never insist upon glasses being worn by a young woman unless you are fully assured that her eyes will suffer harm without them, and then direct that they be worn as little as is positively necessary. Remember that you may impair your patient's general health and happiness more by forcing her to wear glasses than the eyes would suffer without them. These are but brief hints. There are numerous conditions that will come up to exercise your skill and judgment. As to the amount of hyperopia you should correct you must consider all the conditions we have touched upon. In strabismus convergens it is generally well to correct the total hyperopia. As a rule, the manifest hyperopia may be corrected, yet sometimes even this is too much; the power and control of accommodation and convergence is to be considered; also the amount and kind of work the patient does, and whether by night or by day, artificial light requiring stronger glasses than daylight. As a rule, the weakest glass that corrects the trouble is the most comfortable. No hard and fast rule can be laid down, our patients being human beings and not optical instruments.

Myopia: The myopic eye is adapted for diverging rays of light. Such rays are given off, so far as the eye is concerned, by objects situated within fifteen feet. The divergence of the rays increases as the distance of the object from the eye decreases. As a result of this, a myopic eye may have perfect vision at and within a certain distance, and very poor vision beyond this point. The greater the distance of this object from the far point of the eye, the poorer will the vision be. In a case of myopia, it is essential to distinguish between normal or physiological myopia and the pathological variety, as they are two very different troubles. The symptoms of normal myopia may be very slight; in fact, one may live a long life and remain totally unconscious of nearsightedness, seeing very well near-by, while distant objects seem covered by a thin veil or haze, which to the average myope is very agreeable. In other cases, distant vision is so poor that the sufferer can not guide his footsteps, and a few such patients will be found who suffer from headache and other reflex pains. Divergent strabismus sometimes appears in the high grades of normal myopia, especially if the vision of one eye is poor, or if the amount of myopia is much greater in one eye than in the other. The commonest form of myopia is the axial, in which the antero-posterior diameter is longer than that of an emmetropic eye. As a result, the eye appears full and prominent, and it is in this form of myopia that the well-developed and often prominent nasal bridge is noticed. In some myopes convergent strabismus seems to exist, owing to the position of the visual line, which in some cases cuts the cornea to the outer side of its center. The diagnosis of normal myopia is easy. It is made by determining the far point of distinct vision with Snelling's test-type, having the patient read the size of type which forms a visual angle of five minutes. Myopia is also determined and measured by the weakest concave lens that enables the patient to see best when the test object is at least fifteen feet from his eye. The subjective examination should be made in the same way as in hyperopia, but in this case the weakest minus glass will give the amount of manifest myopia. The real myopia is often less than the manifest, on account of the ciliary muscle persisting in a state of tonic contraction during the examination. The true amount of myopia can be measured by objective dioptometry in the manner already indicated, or with greater certainty by paralyzing the accommodation by Hydrobromate of Hyoscine. Normal myopia can be distinguished from the pathological form by the normal appearance of the fundus. The treatment is simply the prescription of the proper glasses to correct the refractive error. These glasses are determined, not only by the amount of myopia, but also by the range of accommodation and acuity of vision possessed by the patient. If his acuity of vision is normal, and his range of accommodation very good — that is, if he can read fine print at or within five inches of his correcting glasses, and do this without undue fatigue for fifteen minutes, it will be well to give him the same glass for near and distant vision. Myopia of less than two dioptres seldom requires glasses for near vision, although sometimes these cases prefer to wear their glasses for all purposes. When the vision is good, and the range of accommodation is poor, you should prescribe a weaker minus glass for near work, or even a convex glass, depending upon the amount of myopia and the range of accommodation. If the acuity of vision and the range of accommodation are poor, you may not be able to prescribe any glasses, as the patient will often see better without them, this being due to the diminution in size of the retinal images which minus lenses cause. Stenopaic spectacles will often give fair vision for near work to these cases, but they are of no value for distant vision, on account of the great restriction of the visual field which they cause.

Pathological myopia is divided into the stationary and progressive forms. The axial forms of these varieties of myopia are distinguished from normal myopia by the presence of a posterior staphyloma. This is due to destructive changes in the sclerotic, choroid and retina at and around the posterior pole of the eye, allowing the eyeball to yield to the intra-ocular pressure. Predisposition to this affection is inherited. It tends to increase in youth, being aggravated by the excessive convergence made necessary by the position of the tar point. Poor health, a stooping position and poor light when working at near-by objects also tend to increase this trouble. The progressive form tends to the destruction of the eyesight by the destructive changes set up in the fundus of the eye. Atrophy of the choroid and retina, fluidity of the vitreous, cataractous changes in the lens, and detachment and hemorrhages of the retina are some of the disastrous results of this form of myopia. The stationary can be distinguished from the progressive form by the edge of the staphyloma being clear cut and the vitreous and lens being normal. In the progressive form the edges of the staphyloma will appear indistinct and irregular. We may also find atrophic spots at and around the staphyloma, which have a tendency to coalesce with it. Any or all the pathological changes we have mentioned may be present. The stationary form may be treated in the same way as normal myopia, observing the same rules for prescribing glasses. Warn your patient against using his eyes when the light is poor, direct him to sit erect when reading; caution him against the excessive use of his eyes for near work, and advise him to take all the out-door exercise possible. In the case of the progressive form, insist upon the patient giving up all near work. If his eyes are sensitive to light, direct him to wear gray glasses when in a strong light. If he has to go about, give him glasses for distant vision, and caution him against using them for near work. Be very careful that these glasses are not too strong. If you observe a tendency to spasm of accommodation, keep the ciliary muscle paralyzed by a weak solution of some mydriatic, and this may be kept up for months, the patient wearing dark glasses while the pupil is dilated. You should also prescribe the indicated remedy. Those that give the best results are Nux vomica, Belladonna, Gelsemium, Aurum muriaticum and Aconite. You should make the patient understand that he has diseased eyes, for it is a common belief among the people that a myopic eye is a strong one. When the trouble is arrested, treat it as a non-progressive case. Curvature myopia occurs in spasm of accommodation and in the early stages of cataract. Its treatment must depend upon the cause. Index myopia may result from iritis, but few cases have been observed. It has been noticed in diabetes. It should be treated as axial myopia, at the same time giving due weight to its cause. Among the subjective symptoms of myopia are dark spots and floating objects before the eyes, also flashes of fire and distortion of objects, pain in the eyes and burning of the lids, with headache and other asthenopic symptoms, though myopes are never so loud in their complaints as are hyperopes. As a rule, you will have no trouble in persuading your myopic patients to wear glasses which enable them to see the world, but there are others who will not wear glasses that make their vision acute, claiming that such acute vision is painful to them and serves to keep them in a nervous and irritable state. Others lament that the glasses have taken away the beautiful hazy world in which they have heretofore lived. Many such patients will throw aside the glasses, preferring to live in their world of diffusion circles.

Astigmatism: The astigmatic eye cannot bring rays of light emanating from a point to a focus on its retina. In other words, homocentric light ceases to be homocentric after refraction. Strictly speaking, this applies only to monochromatic light, as we do not call chromatic aberration of the eye astigmatism. We have treated of three refractive conditions of the eye, emmetropia, hyperopia and myopia. The presence of any two of these refractive conditions, or of an unequal amount of hyperopia or myopia in the several meridians of one eye, will constitute regular astigmatism. In irregular astigmatism we may have any or all and varying amounts of these several refractive conditions in one and the same meridian. In regular astigmatism, while the refractive power of the eye differs in its several meridians, any one meridian will have the same refractive power throughout its extent. The meridians of maximum and minimum refraction are called the principal meridians. These two principal meridians are always at right angles to each other, and are termed the meridians of short and long curvature. In most eyes the vertical meridian has a shorter radius of curvature than has the horizontal, and when this is the case the point of distinct vision for horizontal lines will lie nearer the eye than that for vertical lines. But bear in mind that the principal meridians are not always vertical and horizontal, but may run in any direction, yet are always at right angles with each other. Nearly all eyes are astigmatic. If the amount of astigmatism is slight, so as not to be susceptible of profitable correction, it is called normal astigmatism.

A study of the course of rays of light radiating from a point situated in front of the cornea, after their refraction by the different meridians of the astigmatic eye, will be of great interest and value in explaining the peculiarities of astigmatic vision. The rays of light that pass through the meridians of the shorter radius of curvature will cross each other at a place anterior to the place of crossing of the rays passing through the meridians of the longer radius of curvature. The rays at the place of crossing do not form a point of light, but a luminous line. The direction of these lines is at right angles to the meridians, which cause them to cross. The vertical meridian will form a horizontal line. The length and distance apart of these lines, which are termed the anterior and posterior focal lines, depend upon the difference of refractive power between the two principal meridians of the eye. An eye whose vertical meridian has a shorter radius of curvature than its horizontal meridian (and this is the rule) will have a horizontal line for its anterior focus, and a vertical line for its posterior focus. Now, if the retina is situated at the anterior focal line, the point of light will appear elongated in a horizontal direction. On the other hand, if the retina and posterior focal line correspond, the retinal image of the luminous point will be elongated in a vertical direction. The distance between these two focal lines is termed the focal interval. If the retina were placed midway between the focal lines, the ocular image of the luminous point would be a circle of dispersion. If the retina were anywhere between the anterior focal line and the circle of dispersion, the luminous point would form an oblate ellipse of diffusion. The same would be true if the posterior focal interval was cut, only the ellipse would be prolate. In case the retina was anterior to the anterior focal lines, the form of dispersion would be a large oblate ellipse. If posterior to the posterior focal line, it would be a large prolate ellipse. A line may be conceived to be made up of infinite number of points arranged in such a manner that its length exceeds its breadth several times. The retinal image of a line will undergo the 'same diffusion after refraction by an astigmatic eye that images of points undergo under like conditions. Where the focus of the vertical meridian of the eye and its retina coincide, a point will appear drawn out horizontally. In other words, instead of appearing as a point it will appear as a horizontal line. Under the same condition, a vertical line placed before the eye will appear as a broad, indistinct band, and if there were two lines, separated by a distance equal to their breadth, the dispersion images might overlap to such an extent that they would appear as one wide, indistinct surface. In the case of horizontal lines, we would have the ocular image drawn out in the direction of the length of the line; as a consequence, the line would be elongated and indistinct at its ends. This explanation of the behavior of points and lines will hold, whatever the form of the object may be. The causes of astigmatism may be anatomical or pathological. Among the anatomical causes are: difference in the radii of curvature of the two principal meridians of the cornea, or crystalline lens, or the optical centers of the lens and cornea may be out of line, or the axes of the cornea may not be parallel, or the different sections of the lens may have different curvatures or indices of refraction. Some of the pathological causes are: wounds to the cornea, especially the incisions made in the operation for cataract, or iridectomy, cataractous changes of the lens and ulceration of the cornea.

The most important functional cause is spasmodic contraction of certain sectors of the ciliary muscle. The form of an object is more readily made out from lines of dispersion than from either ellipses or circles of dispersion, and it is for this reason that, when the astigmatic patient can bring either of his focal lines upon his retina, he will see better than with an equal amount of uncorrected myopia or hyperopia. Myopes will often look through their glasses diagonally, if the glasses are too weak to correct their refractive errors, thus rendering themselves astigmatic in order to see better. Patients can correct their astigmatism in several ways. By facing a bright light, or by bringing objects near-by, so causing the pupil to contract, or by nipping the lids together, by rapidly changing the accommodative force as they view different parts of an object, and, in binocular vision, by the union of the two eyes correcting the defect in each. On account of the great power that some astigmatic persons have of correcting their errors of refraction, astigmatism may remain concealed for years. Those who are myopic or hyperopic in the vertical, and emmetropic in the horizontal meridian, can correct their astigmatism by nipping their eyelids, without using their accommodation to obtain distinct vision. If they have hyperopia of unequal degrees in the two meridians, they can overcome it by nipping and accommodating at the same time. If they are myopic in the vertical meridian, and hyperopic in the horizontal, it can be overcome in the same way. About the only form they can not correct, when the principal meridians are vertical and horizontal, is when they are myopic in all meridians in unequal degrees. If the principal meridians are oblique, the patient will often carry his head sideways so as to make the meridians coincide with perpendicular or horizontal objects; but when the principal meridians are oblique, it is not possible for him to correct his vision without the aid of some optical appliance. The amount of astigmatism is determined by finding the difference between the refractive conditions of the different meridians of the eye. It is practical to measure only regular astigmatism. Donders divided regular astigmatism in the following manner:

(1) Simple Myopic and Simple Hyperopic Astigmatism, where there is my-opia or hyperopia in one meridian and emmetropia in the others; they are expressed by the signs Am and Ah.

(2) Compound Myopic and Compound Hyperopic Astigmatism, where there is myopia or hyperopia in all the meridians, but of an unequal amount; they are expressed by the signs M. Am. or H. Ah.

(3) Mixed astigmatism, where there is myopia in one meridian and hyper-opia in the other; this is expressed by the sign Amh. when the myopia pre-dominates, and by the sign Ahm. when the hyperopia predominates.

The diagnosis of astigmatism may be made both subjectively and objec-tively. Each method has its advantages, and neither should be used to the exclusion of the other. Of the subjective methods, the ones of most practical value are the stenopaic slit test, the test by cards of parallel and radiating lines, and the test by cylindrical lenses. An examination combining these three tests will give the most certain and accurate results, and in the long run will be found to be the most rapid way of determining the presence of astig-matism, the direction of the principal meridians of the eye, and the kind and amount of error. To determine astigmatism subjectively, the patient should be placed not less than 5 mm. from Snelling's test-types, as in the examina-tion of other errors of refraction, but in addition to the test letters you will have an "astigmatic chart" hung beside it. Probably the best of these charts is the one having radiating bands of three lines each, each line in a band being of such a breadth as to form an angle of one minute, when placed at the test-ing distance. Like the test letters, these lines should be separated from each other by a space equal to their breadth. You will now direct your patient to read the test type with one eye covered, taking care that the eye being tested is kept opened to its normal extent. The patient must neither nip the lids nor open them wider than is normal. You will note if he reads some of the letters incorrectly while reading other smaller letters accurately, which would be an indication of astigmatism. Now direct his attention to the chart lines, and ask him if he notices any difference in the distinctness of the various bands. The direction of the one he sees most distinctly will be at right angles to the me-ridian of the eye that is adapted to the distance of the test card. As a rule, the horizontal stripes are seen best in hyperopic astigmatism, and the vertical are seen best in myopic astigmatism. This is but a rule, not a law. Now place the stenopaic slit in front of the eye, at right angles to the direction of the band of lines which the patient saw most distinctly, and have him read the test letters. Then rotate the slit in both directions from the first position until you have found the place where he sees the letters most distinctly, and then rotate it at right angles to the position of most distinct vision, and note if his vision is made worse thereby. If you have found a difference in his vision in the different positions of the slit, he is astigmatic. Now try spherical lenses in front of the slit, and note whether they make vision better or worse, in either or both positions of the slit. If a convex lens makes vision better, or if it remains as good, or if it does not make vision worse, and a minus lens does not make vision better, then you have a case of simple hyperopic astigmatism of about the amount of the strongest plus glass that did this. If a convex lens improves or does not make vision worse in both positions, yet he stood a stronger glass in one position than in another, then you have a case of compound hyperopic astigmatism, the difference between the strong and weak lens giving about the amount of astigmatism, the weaker one giving about the amount of hyperopia. If a minus lens in one position of the slit and a plus lens in the other made vision better, then you have a case of mixed astigmatism. If a minus lens made vision better in one direction and not in another, and a plus lens made it worse in the second position of the slit, it is a case of simple myopic astigmatism. If minus lenses improve vision in both positions of the slit, but a stronger lens is required in one position than in another, it is a case of compound myopic astigmatism. If the case is one of hyperopic or myopic astigmatism, take out the slit from the trial frame and place the indicated "cylinder" in the frame, with the axis of the cylinder corresponding to the most emmetropic meridian as ascertained by the stenopaic slit. Rotate the axis of the lens to either side of this meridian to find the position where vision is best. Then try weaker and stronger lenses, rotating their axis, to see if yon can find a position where vision is better. In compound cases you should find the indicated spherical lens in addition to the cylindrical, following the same rule as in simple cases as regards strength and the position of the axis of the cylinder. Having found what seems to be the best combination, try weak plus and minus lenses before it to see if you have over or under corrected the error. In mixed cases place the plus and minus cylinders at right angles to each other, making their axes correspond with the two principal meridians of the eye, the axis of the plus lens in the myopic meridian and the axis of the minus lens in the hyperopic meridian. You will find, as a rule, that the correcting glasses will make vision better than the slit alone, or the slit combined with spherical lenses. This is due to the facts that the slit does not correct all the astigmatism, that it reduces the amount of illumination, and that the diffraction due to the slit reduces vision by blurring. Having made the test for astigmatism at a distance, and recorded it, you should then try the glasses which give the best vision for reading and other near work. Of the objective tests for astigmatism, you are already familiar with the one made with the ophthalmoscope. The only other one we will mention is the one made with the ophthalmometer. This instrument measures the radii of curvature of the cornea for an area of about 5 mm. in diameter. It is of use in determining the approximate amount of corneal astigmatism, and in giving the axis of maximum and minimum refraction of that membrane. In mixed astigmatism the ophthalmometer is of no value. The eye must be kept fully opened when using the ophthalmometer, as pressure on the cornea will cause its curvature to vary. The great objection to the use of this instrument for practical purposes, when used alone, is that we can not be sure that it gives the true amount of astigmatism. For this reason tests by it must always be supplemented by other tests. This is in a measure true of all tests, both subjective and objective. The action of the ciliary muscle may falsify all the subjective tests, and the inability to measure the patient's vision objectively often renders the objective tests worthless. When to paralyze the accommodation is determined by the agreement or lack of agreement of the subjective and objective tests. When the subjective test, as we have given it, and the objective tests, by direct ophthalmoscopy and skiascopy are in perfect agreement you need not, as a rule, paralyze the accommodation. When the tests are not in agreement, more especially if the error seems to be of the myopic form, it becomes necessary to paralyze the accommodation. When an astigmatic patient should wear glasses will depend upon the amount and kind of astigmatism, the direction of the principal meridians, the amount of asthenopia, and upon the kind and amount of work he has to do. His age should also be taken into consideration. The simple and compound hyperopic astigmatics will be compelled to wear their glasses more than those suffering from simple myopic astigmatism. The compound myopic astigmatics will be compelled to use glasses whenever they wish to see distinctly at a distance.

Irregular astigmatism is divided into normal and abnormal. The normal form is due to the structure of the lens. The abnormal is due to irregularities of the cornea, or lens, or of both. The acuteness of vision is but slightly decreased by ordinary normal irregular astigmatism. Abnormal irregular astigmatism causes a very great impairment of vision, even if the defect is very slight. Anything that causes irregularity of curvature, or of the structure of the cornea, or of the lens, will give rise to irregular astigmatism. The diagnosis of irregular astigmatism is established if the stenopaic hole improves vision when all other means fail to improve it. It is seldom practical to grind a glass to correct irregular astigmatism, although stenopaic spectacles will often give good practical vision for near work.

Anisometropia: A difference in the refractive power of the two eyes is termed anisometropia. One eye may be emmetropic and the other hyperopic, myopic or astigmatic, or both may be hyperopic, myopic or astigmatic, but in different degrees. Any case in which the refractive conditions of the two eyes are found to be at variance would be a case of anisometropia. In anisometropia the patient may have binocular vision; he may have vision with each of the eyes alternately, or he may use only one eye and exclude the other. The treatment of anisometropia will depend upon the amount of difference, the kind of difference, the range of accommodation, the presence or absence of binocular vision, and the power the patient may have of mentally fusing two dissimilar images. In prescribing glasses for this condition, always correct the best eye when it is not practical to correct both. Where the eyes are astigmatic, you can, as a rule, correct them both. When one is emmetropic and the other ametropic, they are better off without glasses for distant vision. When both are myopic or hypermetropic, you can generally correct both if the difference is not greater than two dioptres, and if the range of accommodation is good. If one eye is hyperopic and the other is myopic, you may correct one, or both, or neither, or sometimes the patient will do better with both partly corrected. If there is a great difference in the size of the ocular images, the patient will seldom stand full correction. For example, with aphakia in one eye and myopia in the other, you should not attempt to correct both eyes if he has binocular vision and his sight is good in each eye after correction.

Have the patient try the glasses for distant and near vision with both eyes separately and together, asking him to describe the apparent size of the object. If there is a great difference in the apparent size of the object as seen by the two eyes, then you must test several times over before giving him glasses.

Presbyopia: This term signifies inability to read fine type at a distance of eight French inches from the eye, and that this inability is due to senile changes in the eye. The term is an arbitrary one, and the distance at which fine type should be read was proposed by Donders. The failure of accommodation as life advances is very constant, being first noticed after the tenth year.

The following table shows the range of accommodation corresponding to the different ages:

Years.	Dioptres.
10	14
15	12
20	10
25	8.5
30	7
35	5.5
40	4.5
45	3.5
50	2.5
55	1.75
60	1.
65	.75
70	.25
75	0

Keep a copy of this table upon your trial case, as it will prove a great help in selecting glasses for near vision. A myopic eye of less than eight inches will never become presbyopic. Myopes, whose far point is less than eight inches, and all persons who are emmetropic, hyperopic or astigmatic, will become presbyopic as age advances. In emmetropic persons, presbyopia is generally established about the fortieth year.

Hyperopes will have to wear stronger glasses to correct their presbyopia than will emmetropes, while myopes will require weaker ones for the same purpose. From these facts we deduce the following rule for prescribing glasses for presbyopia: Add the amount of hyperopia to the amount of presbyopia, or subtract the amount of myopia from the presbyopia. This rule will also' apply to all forms of regular astigmatism complicated with presbyopia. The term premature presbyopia is often used to designate paralysis of accommodation. In prescribing glasses for presbyopia, you must not attempt to make all your patients see at eight inches; but you must find the region in which they wish to accommodate, and prescribe the glass that enables them to work comfortably within that region. Most patients have a dread of glasses too strong, and, while glasses that are too strong may not hurt the eyes, they do shorten the region of accommodation and often cause pain and annoyance. It is true such glasses will last longer, but this should be a small consideration with most patients. From forty to fifty years of age the glasses should be changed every year or two. From fifty to sixty-five every two years, and from sixty-five onward one pair may last five or ten years.

Chapter Twelve - Diseases of the Lens

Diseases of the lens and its capsule are included under the general term cataract. Of inflammations of the lens (phakitis) we know nothing, though the proliferation of the cells lining the posterior surface of the anterior capsule, occurring in capsular cataract, seems to approach this condition. The term cataract, is applied to opacities of the lens or its capsule. The two primary divisions of cataract are lenticular and capsular. They are termed lenticular when the substance of the lens is the seat of the opacity, and capsular when the capsule is opaque, though in reality the opacity does not reside in the capsule, but in a layer of new-formed tissue (which bears a resemblance to connective tissue) intimately in contact with the posterior surface of the anterior capsule, and in the remains of the hyaloid artery, which causes an opacity on the posterior surface of the posterior capsule. When both the lens substance and the capsule are opaque, the condition is called capsulo-lenticular cataract. The sub-divisions of cataract are many, viz.: Nuclear and cortical, hard and soft, circumscribed and diffuse, progressive and stationary, idiopathic and traumatic, congenital, acquired, senile, simple, complicated, etc., etc. The subjective symptoms of uncomplicated cataract are dimness of vision, which may be very slight or amount to practical blindness, though the light sense is never completely lost, and muscae voliantes, or specks in the field of vision, and polyopia monocularis, or multiple vision of single objects. The objective symptoms consist of changes in the transparency of the lens and its capsules, the opacities appearing grayish by reflected and black by transmitted light. Opacities of the anterior capsule, or marked ones of the lens within the pupillary space, may be recognized by ordinary light, the pupil appearing gray, the shade of which may vary from almost white in the capsular and very soft lenticular cataracts to very dark yellowish gray where the nucleus and cortex are involved. Oblique illumination and dilatation of the pupil may bring into view minute opacities, appearing as striae, sectors,, disks, spindles, etc. By illumination of the eye with the ophthalmoscopic mirror, the opacities that appeared gray by reflected light will appear black. The pathology of cataract will be given under each special form. The senile is the most common form, and in it the more central part of the lens, called the nucleus, becomes sclerosed, and, as it shrinks, spaces form between it and the cortical part. These spaces become filled with fluid, whose index of refraction diners from the rest of the lens; this in itself would give rise to opacity, but added to this are opacities of the cortex, which may be mainly around the nucleus, where the term nuclear cataract would be applied. The opacities may take the form of s. riae or sectors which may be few in number and limited to any part of the cortex. They may be in the pupillary area or concealed by the iris. Punctate or irregularly-shaped spots of opacity may appear, or a cloud-like opacity, may be present. The more circumscribed the opacity the less the interference with vision. The more diffuse and the more centrally located, the more they impair sight. When the cortex becomes completely opaque, the cataract is said to be ripe and ready for operation. This condition is determined by the absence of shadow when light is thrown obliquely upon the iris. The way to detect the shadow of the iris in the lens is to concentrate the light from a flame, by means of a convex lens, and throw it obliquely into the eye. The more transparent the lens substance intervening between the posterior surface of the iris and the opacity, the broader will be the shadow. The term cataract dura, or hard cataract, is also applied to senile cataracts. Most senile cataracts are mixed in character, being partly nuclear and partly cortical. There is a form of senile cataract in which the whole lens becomes sclerosed, appearing like a large nucleus. This form never becomes ripe in the sense of becoming completely opaque, for while it may be of an amber color, or sometimes almost black, it remains more or less transparent, though the vision may be so reduced that the patient can not do more than count fingers at a few feet from the eye. When only a few opaque striae, or very faint, cloud-like opacities, exist in the lens, the cataract is called incipient. When further advanced, it is called immature; and when the lens is completely opaque the cataract is said to be mature or ripe. Hyper-mature and morgagnian are terms that are applied to a cataract in which the cortical substance has become fluid. Disintegration and absorption may be carried to such an extent that the fluid may become transparent, and the sclerosed nucleus may be detected floating in it. After a great length of time even the nucleus may disintegrate. In hyper-mature cataract, with oblique illumination, the nucleus can be seen as an amber-colored body, which changes its position with the movements of the eye. Senile cataract is a progressive affection, sometimes progressing very slowly and sometimes very rapidly. Again, there will be periods when it becomes stationary, and the lens even seems to grow more transparent, after which the lens becomes rapidly opaque. The more diffuse the opacity and the nearer the nucleus it is, the more rapid is the progress of the cataract. The more circumscribed the opacity, and the nearer the periphery the slower will be the growth of the cataract. Medicines seem to exert very little action in clearing a lens that has become opaque. In the earlier stages, it has seemed to me that they hold the progress of the disease in check. The remedy that has given me the most satisfaction is Nux vom. 3x, a tablet every day, continued indefinitely. When the cataract becomes sufficiently opaque to make the patient practically blind, it should be removed. This stage of maturity is the best time for its removal. It is very difficult to completely remove an immature cataract, for some of the cortical substance adheres to the capsule, absorbs the aqueous humor and becomes opaque, at the same time setting up a hyperplasia of the cells of the capsule, resulting in a thick opaque membrane which is called a secondary cataract. Then a second operation is necessary to make an opening through this opaque membrane. (For removal of cataract, see chapter on Operations.)

Of the circumscribed cataracts there are many varieties. Anterior polar cataract generally occurs in children, as a result of a perforation of the cornea from ulceration. The apex of the lens striking the posterior surface of the cornea with some violence causes a disturbance of the capsular cells at that point, the result being a circumscribed capsular cataract. If the opaque portion projects above the plane of the rest of the capsule, it is termed pyramidal cataract. These are generally small and interfere very little with vision unless the pupil is exceedingly small. As a rule, the condition is not recognized until all the tissue changes due to the injury have passed. Treatment will be of no avail, and an operation is not justifiable.

Posterior polar cataract is due to the remnants of the hyaloid artery, causing an opacity on the posterior capsule. If the opacity is small, it will not cause much diminution of visual acuity. It should be let alone.

Zonular or lamellar cataract is characterized by the lens being transparent in its center, which is surrounded by a layer of opaque lens substance, this again being surrounded by transparent lens tissue. The opacity is supposed to occur in early childhood, in badly nourished subjects, and as a result of convulsions. The circumscribed forms are stationary. There is a form with opaque radii running from the shell-like central opacity, and, as a rule, this form is stationary. The treatment is to open a pathway for rays of light to enter the eyeball. This may be done in two ways. If the opacity is small and nonprogressive, an iridectomy will be the best operation. If large, a discussion. (See Operations.)

Anterior and posterior polar cataracts are often the result of traumatism, or of a diseased condition of other parts of the eye. They are characterized by the opacity being within the lens tissue, near the anterior or posterior capsule. Their treatment would depend upon the cause. If the lens become entirely opaque, removal is the only treatment. The general diseases which sometimes cause cataract are diabetes and nephritis. Cataracts have been produced, experimentally, in rabbits by naphthalin. Severe cold and lightning-stroke have been known to cause the development of cataract. Traumatic cataracts are generally due to a rupture of the capsule, which admits the aqueous humor, and this causes the cortical substance to swell and become opaque. If the rupture in the capsule is very small, the opacity may be limited to the immediate vicinity of the injury. If the rupture is large, the whole lens will become opaque, and it may swell very rapidly, causing an increase of tension in the eyeball with all its attending dangers.

Treatment: If the patient is seen immediately after the injury, put him to bed and have the eye kept cold by the application of iced cloths. Give Aconite

1x, a tablet every hour. If symptoms of iritis develop, keep the pupil dilated. If the lens swells very rapidly, and the eyeball becomes hard, an iridectomy should be made at once and the lens matter removed. Complicated cataracts are to be diagnosed by the existence of other diseases. Calcareous and cholesterine deposits are sometimes found in cataractous lenses. Before advising or undertaking the removal of a cataract, the field of vision for light perception should be examined, and if the patient can not correctly locate the flame of a candle, held about two feet in front of him, in all parts of the visual field, then suspect some disease of the deeper structures that might make an operation inadvisable. Cataracts in young children should be operated as soon as possible, otherwise the retina may lose its functional power from disuse. In adults, if one eye is cataractous and the sight of the other is good, there need be no hurry about operating; at the same time it should not be allowed to become over-ripe. After the removal of a cataract the patient will have to wear glasses to enable him to see distinctly, as he will have lost the power of accommodation. He will probably need two pairs, one for distant and one for near vision. He can gain a certain amount of accommodation by sliding his glasses up and down his nose; as a rule, a given plus lens will become weaker as the spectacles approach the eye and stronger as they recede. The glasses should not be given too soon after an operation, not sooner than two months, nor should the eye be used to any extent before that time. The vision will go on improving for several weeks after the operation. Before operating on any one for cataract, warn him that, while the great majority of operations result in restoration of vision, some are failures.

Dislocations of the lens: Luxation of the lens may be partial or complete. The incomplete form may consist of a mere turning of the lens on its axis. Luxations may be congenital or acquired. The congenital displacements are generally upwards, or upwards and inwards, or upwards and outwards. The cause of dislocation of the lens is either weakness or rupture of the zonule of Ziun. The luxated lens may be either transparent or opaque. Upon dilatation of the pupil, the extent of displacement of the opaque lens may be easily made out; the part of the pupil not occupied by the lens will appear black, while that part which is occupied by it will appear gray. If the lens be transparent, the part of the pupil free from the lens will appear of a darker black than the other parts. By reflected light the edge of the lens will appear very bright, owing to total reflection of the light. By transmitted light (ophthahnoscopic examination) the edge will appear black, the light from the fundus not passing through this part of the lens owing to total reflection.

Traumatic displacements may vary from a slight turning of the lens to complete expulsion from the eyeball, or lodgment under the conjunctiva.

Dislocation may be posterior, into the vitreous, or anterior, into the anterior chamber. Dislocation into the anterior chamber is a very dangerous condition, and demands removal at once, there being great danger of glaucoma, iridocyclitis or keratitis being set up (remove as a senile cataract). Slight luxations had best be let alone unless the lens becomes opaque; then treat them as cataracts. Nothing can be done for a lens dislocated into the vitreous. It may remain for a long time without causing trouble, but sooner or later it will probably cause a cyclitis that will produce blindness. Owing to the loss of support when the lens is luxated, the iris will become tremulous; this condition is called iridodonesis. Dislocation always causes some impairment of sight, either on account of astigmatism, or hyperopia, or myopia, as any or all of these conditions may be caused by dislocation of the lens.

The glass that is found by experiment to give the best vision should be prescribed, unless it causes confusion and interferes with binocular vision.

Lenticonus is a rare anomaly.

In the lens of old people a ring of grayish opacity is often found, generally about the equator. It is called the arcus senilis lentis. It shows very little tendency to spread and should not be mistaken for a cataract.

Diseases of the Vitreous.

Hyalitis is the term applied to inflammation of the vitreous, though simple hyalitis is something we know very little about, foreign bodies in the vitreous being in all probability the most frequent cause. The great majority of diseases of the vitreous are secondary to disease of the ciliary body, choroid or retina. The subjective symptoms of abnormalities of the vitreous are impairment of vision, which may vary from a slight haze to a complete loss of sight, or a variation in the amount of vision from one minute to another, or the presence of specks or floating objects in the field of vision. These specks are called muscae voliantes, and may be pathological or normal. The pathological cause of this condition is opaque bodies in the vitreous, and they may be discovered objectively during life. The normal muscae are caused by the remnants of transparent cells and shreds of membrane, the index of refraction of which differs from that of the surrounding vitreous, casting shadows on the retina. These cells and shreds of membrane may be discovered by the microscope after death. The objective symptom is total opacity of the vitreous, when, no matter how much light is thrown in the eye, none returns to the observer. This condition is generally due to hemorrhage into the vitreous from some of the intra-ocular vessels. If the amount of hemorrhage is slight and is confined to the more anterior parts of the vitreous, a red reflex may be obtained by oblique illumination.

Diffuse haziness is a condition which exists when the light from the vitreous is reflected irregularly and there are no particles in the vitreous of a sufficient size to be seen as forms. This condition may occur in diseases of the ciliary body, choroid or retina.

Dust-like opacities can be best made out by feeble illumination from a plane mirror, or a concave one can be used by reducing the amount of incident light. A strong convex lens should be placed behind the sight hole of the ophthalmoscope to magnify the specks. These are said to be characteristic symptoms of central syphilitic retinitis. The larger opacities, with the exception of the remnants of the hyaloid artery, are generally the result of some past inflammation, or of a hemorrhage that has been partly absorbed. These opacities may be stationary or floating. The rapidity of their motion indicates the fluidity of the vitreous. The opacity due to the remnants of the hyaloid artery presents the form of an opaque line running from the optic disk towards the lens, the posterior surface of which it may reach. Fluidity of the vitreous is termed synchisis. It is the result of disorganization, but is sometimes found without other evidence of ocular disease. Synchisis scintillans is due to the presence of cholesterine crystals in the vitreous, which shine and sparkle when light is thrown upon them. The cause of this trouble is unknown, and it gives rise to very little disturbance. The amount of disturbance of vision caused by opacities of the vitreous varies with the position and kind of opacity. The more central the situation the greater the disturbance. A small, dense opacity will not cause as much disturbance of vision as will a large, transparent one.

We distinguish opacities of the vitreous from those in the posterior part of the lens by noting the direction of movement of the opacity. If its movement is with that of the eye, the opacity must be anterior to the center of rotation, which is just posterior to the lens, and therefore the opacity is in the lens. If the opacity is behind the center of rotation (in the vitreous), it will, of course, move in the opposite direction to the movement of the front part of the eye. The deeper it lies in the vitreous the greater excursion will it make with a given movement of the eyeball. In synchisis the tension of the eyeball is decreased, and often the zonule of Zinn becomes weakened, iridodonesis results; the presence of this symptom, in the absence of dislocation of the lens, indicates synchisis, and it may be our only guide to diagnosis if the lens is opaque or if there are no opacities in the vitreous.

Foreign bodies in the vitreous are very apt to be followed by severe inflammatory symptoms, though sometimes they become encapsulated, and remain for years without producing symptoms other than a break in the field of vision.

Yet they are always a source of danger, and should be removed at once, if possible. Of all foreign bodies pieces of iron are the most easy to remove. A magnet for this purpose may be introduced into the vitreous, either through the opening made by the passage of the piece of iron, or through a new opening, if one can be made without involving the ciliary body. Other foreign bodies can sometimes be seized with a fine pair of forceps, or by a hook, and so removed. Entozoa of the vitreous, are of exceeding great rarity in this country. Suppuration of the vitreous occurs in panophthalmitis. It presents a distinct yellowish opacity when viewed by the ophthalmoscope.

Circumscribed exudations in the vitreous may be mistaken for glioma, but the history of the case and the lack of increase of tension will assist in diagnosis. (See Glioma.) Prognosis of opacities of the vitreous will depend upon the condition that produced them, and whether recent or of long standing.

Hamamelis θ is the best remedy in hemorrhage into the vitreous.

Thuja θ, Kali iod. 1x, Merc, biniod. 3x, Merc. corr. 3x, and Hepar sulph. 3x, when the opacities are diffuse. (For detailed symptoms and other remedies, see Diseases of the Ciliary Body, Choroid and Retina.)

Diseases of the Choroid.

Diseases of the choroid may be divided into three groups. The first, includeing all the diseases that do not tend to suppurate; the second, including all the suppurative forms; and the third, all the tumors of the choroid. The first group may be subdivided into the diseases in which the inflammatory symptoms predominate, and into those in which the predominate symptoms are those of degeneration. Disseminated, central, aureolar and syphilitic choroiditis are distinct clinical types of inflammatory disease of the choroid. Disseminated choroiditis may present no extra-ocular evidence of its existence. There is no pain if the inflammation is limited to the choroid. There may be a very slight or a very great impairment of vision, depending upon the part of the choroid affected and upon the condition of the vitreous and lens. An ophthalmoscopic examination in the early stages may reveal a transparent or a more or less opaque vitreous. Both the direct and indirect methods should be used in making an intraocular examination in this disease. The indirect method for making a general examination, and the direct method to study the details and to examine the

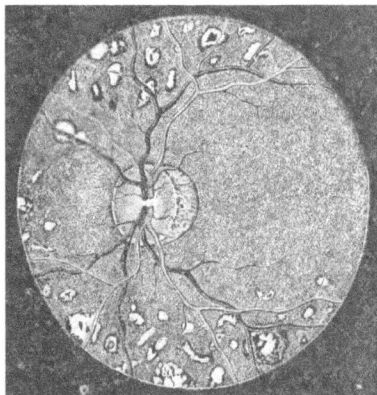

Choroiditis Disseminata. (After De Wecker.)

vitreous. If the vitreous is sufficiently transparent to permit of a distinct view of the fundus, there may be seen, during the early stages of the disease, pale yellow spots. These spots are not confined to any one part of the fundus, but, as a rule, they are most frequently found in the equatorial region; sometimes they are limited to the most anterior part of the choroid, and in this case may be readily overlooked. In order to see them, direct the patient to look up and down, to the right and to the left, then up and to the right, up and to the left, down and to the right, then down and to the left; this will bring all the peripheral parts of the choroid into view. These spots may vary in size from one-fourth that of the disk to three or four times the disk diameter. Their outlines are very apt to be indistinct, and they occupy a plane posterior to the retinal vessels, which may be often seen passing over them. This distinguishes them from retinal exudation. The color presented by the spot in the

114

early stage is due (aside from the color of the light used for the examination) to the color of the exudation, the layer of the choroid in which it lies, the amount of pigment contained in the pigment layer of the retina, and to the amount of displacement of the pigment cells of this layer. In the late or atrophic stage of the disease the spots may be yellowish white, white or bluish white, sometimes with a border of black pigment, sometimes with masses of pigment scattered over them. Their shape may be circular, oval or very irregular, and their outlines are generally well defined. In the larger spots choroidal vessels are sometimes seen crossing them. These spots of atrophic choroid are to be distinguished from retinal exudations by the fact that the retinal vessels may be seen passing over them. The retinal exudations are very apt to cover the vessels at some point of their course. The color of the atrophic spots is due to the more or less complete destruction of the choroidal tissue, and to the absorption of certain portions of the pigment layer of the retina, and to an increase and heaping up of pigment in the other parts of the pigment layer. If a certain amount of the choroidal tissue remains, the spot will appear of a yellowish white color. If it has been replaced by a certain amount of cicatricial tissue, the color will be white. If the destruction of the choroidal tissue has been complete, so that the sclera adheres directly to the retina, the color will be a bluish white.

Hemorrhage from the choroidal vessels is very rare in this disease. Hyperaemia of the disk or retina may be present in the very early stages of the disease, and may be the cause of mistakes in diagnosis. Iritis sometimes exists as a complication. In the late stages synchisis or cataract may be observed.

Pathology: Disseminated, inflammatory foci are the peculiarity of this disease. The changes that take place in these foci consist of inflammatory exudation, with proliferation of the cellular elements of the choroid, the formation of young, fibrous stroma, and the destruction of the choroidal stroma and the smaller vessels and capillaries. As a result of these changes, and the subsequent contraction of the new formed cicatricial tissue, changes are set up in the posterior layers of the retina which overlie and surround the destroyed choroidal area. This atrophy of the posterior layer of the retina results in the loss of that part of sight in the visual field corresponding to the part of the retina affected. This blank in the visual field is called Scotoma. In the early stages of retinal destruction the patient may be conscious of a grayish opacity in the visual field (more especially if the macula lutea is affected). This condition would be called a positive scotoma. When this opacity disappears, and the patient sees nothing in that part of his visual field, it simply appearing as a gap in the field, the term negative scotoma is applied. When the disease of the choroid has been very extensive a yellow atrophy of the optic disk results, probably brought about by the destruction of the ganglionic cells of the retina. This is known as choroidal atrophy of the optic nerve. The synchisis and opacity of the vitreous are, in all probability, the result of malnutrition. When we consider that the choroid is essentially a vascular membrane, and also that the hemorrhage is exceedingly rare, in spite of the vascular destruction, it seems reasonable to believe that disseminated choroiditis starts as an arteritis obliterans.

Etiology, Course, Prognosis and Treatment. — Syphilis, either inherited or acquired, seems to be the most frequent cause. The disease may run its course in utero. When due to acquired syphilis, it generally appears as one of the late secondary symptoms, persons of middle age being the most frequent sufferers. The disease may extend over many months, and relapses are not infrequent, even after several years. The prognosis depends upon the part of the fundus affected; the nearer the macula, the less is the hope of a restoration of useful vision. The earlier the disease is brought under treatment, the greater is the hope of arresting its progress.

Treatment: Protect the eyes from strong light by smoke-colored glasses; keep the patient in the open air as much as possible; direct him to be well fed with good nourishing food and to sleep in a dry, well-ventilated room. Merc, biniod. 3x, a grain tablet three times a day, continued for a long time, will be found to be the best remedy when the vitreous is clear. Thuja, 1x, a drop three times a day (also for a long time), when the vitreous is hazy. Kali iod. 1x, five grains three times a day, when the iris or ciliary body is affected. Merc. corr. 3x, Hepar sulph. 3x, or Bell, 1x, if the retina is affected. (See Diseases of the Retina.) Nux vom. 1x, a grain tablet three times a day, will be found of great value in improving the acuity of vision after the subsidence of the inflammatory symptoms.

Central choroiditis is a variety of the disseminated form, which is limited to the central part of the fundus. It either appears as a single center of inflammation, or as several foci packed closely together. On account of its location it is a much graver trouble as regards sight than the ordinary disseminated form. A scotoma may be the only subjective symptom, at first positive, later negative. By ophthalmoscopic examination the disease will be seen to be limited to the macular region of the fundus. It is to be distinguished from a hemorrhage of the macula, which is not uncommon in this region, by its color, which has already been described under disseminated choroiditis. The color of the hemorrhage, when recent, is of a brighter red than the rest of the fundus. When it is undergoing fatty degeneration it is of a glistening white color. The last stages of the destructive changes set up by the hemorrhage can not be distinguished from those due to central choroiditis. The treatment should be that of disseminated choroiditis, only greater care should be taken to protect the eye from light, and the patient should be impressed with the gravity of the affection. Areolar choroiditis is a form of disseminated choroiditis, that differs from the common variety in being located around the macula lutea, and the spots of exudation are, as a rule, better defined in the early stages than are those of the ordinary form. The final stages also differ, the pigment often being spread over the inflammatory spot; later on the pigment disappears from the center of the spot, leaving a more or less white disk, bordered by a ring of pigment. The prognosis is better than in the common forms of disseminated choroiditis, as there does not seem to be as great an amount of destruction of retinal tissue or of cicatricial contraction.

The pathological changes, especially in the later stages of the disease, bear a close analogy to the disseminated form. The course of the disease is about the same as a mild disseminated case, and the treatment would be the same.

Syphilitic choroido-retinitis. — In all forms of plastic choroiditis the posterior layers of the retina are more or less implicated. In this form the retina seems to be implicated from the start, the symptoms of retinal inflammation being so marked that the disease was formerly described as syphilitic retinitis. The characteristic symptoms are a peculiar form of opacity of the vitreous humor, this structure seeming to be filled with dust, which can be best seen by illuminating the eye with a plane mirror. A concave mirror may be used for the same purpose by turning the light very low. If the eye is moved rapidly up and down several times, and then allowed to rest, the dots in the vitreous may be seen to settle, and in a short time the upper part of the vitreous will look clearer than the lower part. If the vitreous is sufficiently clear to permit of an examination of the retina, the part of it surrounding the optic disk, and extending for some distance along the retinal vessels, will present a pearl grayish haze. The disk is very apt to be redder than normal. The amount of opacity of the vitreous may vary to a great extent, even in the space of twenty-four hours. These may be the only objective symptoms. The subjective symptoms are a great variation in the amount of vision from time to time, flashes of light (phosphenes), objects look distorted (metamorphopsia), or objects look smaller than normal (micropsia). The patient requires a very bright light to see at all well. As evening comes on, and the light diminishes, his sight grows exceedingly poor. This disease is very apt to run a chronic course, and relapses are to be looked for. It may terminate without leaving any trace, or with atrophy of the central part of the choroid and retina, resembling a central choroiditis, or the atrophic spots may resemble those found in disseminated choroiditis, or the fundus may bear a close resemblance to retinitis pigmentosa, and sometimes can be distinguished from it only by the appearance of some change in the choroid and by the history of the case. (See Retinitis Pigmentosa.) Another termination may be atrophy of the optic nerve, or the formation of large membranous opacities in the vitreous, which seem to spring from the optic disk. The cause is syphilis.

Treatment: Protect the eye from bright light, and see that the patient is well fed. Merc. corr. 3x, a grain three times a day, when the vitreous is not very hazy and the outlines of the disk and retinal vessels are indistinct. Kali iod. 1x, a grain three times a day, when the vitreous is hazy and there is difficulty in making out the details of the fundus, especially if the opacities are of perceptible size. Merc, biniod. 2x, a tablet three times a day, if the exudations are to be seen in the choroid, more particularly in the peripheral parts.

Choroidal Degeneration.

Among the affections of the choroid that are of so low a grade as to resemble degenerations rather than inflammations, the one of greatest importance to the practising physician is what has been variously denominated Sclero-Choroiditis Posterior, Staphyloma Posticum, Progressive Myopia, Malignant Myopia, etc. This trouble seems to be a disease of youth, as it makes most rapid progress during that period. In the early stages it manifests itself by the appearance of a white crescent, more or less perfectly shaped, at the outer side of the optic disk. If the disease is progressing, the outlines of the crescent will be irregular and poorly defined; if stationary, the edges will be clear cut and bordered with a more or less perfect line of pigment. The pathological changes are a degeneration and atrophy of the choroid, with a thinning of the sclera and an atrophy of the pigment layer of the retina. This softening of the coats of the eye seems to be confined to the region of the optic nerve and macula lutea, the atrophic crescent often changing to an irregular circle which completely surrounds the disk; but its broadest margin is always towards the macula lutea, though it seldom or ever involves it by direct extension, but it frequently joins other atrophic spots that form in the macular region. The first stages in the formation of atrophic spots in the macular region are a thinning of the retinal pigment, characterized by the appearance of yellowish white streaks. As the disease progresses the spots grow larger and hemorrhages take place, followed by a hazy condition of the surrounding retina, and by opacities of the vitreous. The softening of the ocular coats and the intra-ocular tension lead to a bulging of the posterior part of the eyeball, thus forming a condition termed posterior staphyloma, or ectasia. The formation of a posterior staphyloma will change the refractive condition of the eye. If it were originally hyperopic, it will become emmetropic, then myopic, and the myopia will increase with the growth of the staphyloma.

It is for that reason that the condition has been called progressive or malignant myopia. If the trouble is not arrested, synchisis, posterior polar cataract and detachment of the retina are very likely to occur. The pathological changes that cause the formation of posterior staphyloma are a cause of, and are caused by, pathological myopia.

The primary cause of this trouble we do not know. There may be an inherited weakness of the sclerotic that allows it to yield to the normal intra-ocular pressure, and the consequent stretching may cause the choroid to atrophy and lead to further softening of the sclerotic, and, as a consequence, to further stretching, and so on. Or it may be that a low grade of sclero-choroiditis is the primary condition. But this much we do know, malnutrition of the body, combined with overuse of the eyes for near work, with a poor, dim light, tend to increase the trouble. Upon these facts we base our treatment, which should be rest for the eyes and protection from over-bright light by the use of dark glasses. Work of any kind that demands close mental application, or demands vision at a near point, should be forbidden. The patient should be encouraged to spend a large part of his time in the open air, and he should be well fed and systematically exercised. If a child, he should be taken from school immediately. (For the correction of the refractive defect, see Myopia. For the correction of muscular defects see chapter on Muscles.) Formerly the muscles were supposed to play a great part in progressive myopia; and there is no doubt but that the struggle to maintain binocular vision, under unfavorable conditions, will tend to increase the trouble. Nux vom. 1x, a tablet three times a day, will be found a good remedy to relieve the subjective symptoms and improve the acuity of vision, and it seems to exert a great power in arresting the progress of the disease.

Senile Central Choroiditis belongs to the group in which the symptoms of degeneration are more marked than are those of inflammation. A yellow-red patch appears in the region of the macula; it may be a little larger or smaller than the optic disk, while its outlines are partly regular, it is somewhat difficult to make out, on account of the slight difference in color between it and the surrounding retina, and also on account of its location.

As the pupils of old persons are nearly always small, dilation, by means of some mydriatic, will be found necessary in order to see this trouble distinctly at the early stage Later the choroidal tissue seems to atrophy, and the spot becomes bordered with pigment and is more or less irregular. The symptoms are dimness of vision and distortion of objects, and finally extinction of central vision; but fortunately the disease does not tend to spread beyond the region of the macula. I know of no treatment.

Metastatic choroiditis and panophthalmitis are both forms of suppurative inflammation of the choroid. Panophthalmitis is the common variety, and is most frequently the result of injuries to the anterior part of the eye. Septic infection of the wound is, without doubt, one of the principal factors. The disease is one of the dreaded results of unfortunate cataract operation. The suppuration is never limited to the choroid, but involves all the tissues of the eye. The symptoms are very violent and the disease runs a very rapid course, the eye frequently being destroyed in a single day. Violent pain, with great swelling of the ocular conjunctiva, a hazy state of the cornea, protrusion of the eyeball from swelling of Tenon's capsule, with oedema of the eyelids, are among the first symptoms; these are quickly followed by hypopion and destruction of the cornea. A rupture of the eyeball, with discharge of the contained pus, may give relief; but in any case, after a period of great suffering, the eye shrinks and becomes a worthless stump, which later on may be removed. After panophthalmitis has become established there is no hope of saving the sight. Hepar sulph. 3x should be given every hour. Warm applications should be made, and if the pain is very great an incision involving the anterior part of the sclera, the lens and cornea should be made, so as to give free vent to the pus in the posterior part of the eye. In the early stages, before the suppuration has reached the choroid, the disease may be arrested by having the injury washed thoroughly with a one ten-thousandth solution of Mercurius corrosivus, and give Rhus tox. 3x, every hour, if there is great oedema of the lids and ocular conjunctiva. If hypopion has formed, Hepar sulph. 3x will be the remedy, a tablet every hour. Metastatic choroiditis accompanies grave constitutional diseases, such as puerperal fever, scarlet fever, small-pox, meningitis, typhoid fever, etc. Iritis nearly always occurs as a complication. The treatment is that of the general disease; in addition, a solution of Atropia should be dropped between the eyelids, to keep the pupil dilated. The disease is generally confined to one eye, and may be arrested in any stage. The localized forms that are sometimes seen in children may be mistaken for glioma; indeed, the disease is often called false glioma. It is to be distinguished from the true by the presence of synechia, and by the tension of the eyeball, which is generally decreased; and by the appearance of the mass within the eyeball, being generally flatter and less vascular than the glioma; nor does it tend to increase in size, but there are many cases where it is impossible to distinguish between the two without waiting too long a time. When in doubt, it is wiser to remove the eye if it has no sight. (See Glioma.)

Tubercles of the choroid appear as pale, rose-colored, illy-defined spots, situated, as a rule, around the optic disk. They may be so small as to be just visible, or several millimetres in diameter, or of any size between these extremes. Their appearance is generally an indication of a fatal termination of the general disease. The treatment should be directed to the general trouble.

Tumors of the choroid are generally sarcomatous, either pigmented or non-pigmented. The diagnosis is determined by the presence of a tumor, an increase of tension, and tendency of the vessels upon the growth to appear very prominent. Enucleation of the eyeball is the proper treatment, and this should be done at the earliest possible date. If the tumor has broken through the eyeball and involved the orbital tissues, the entire contents of the orbit should be removed, and the periosteum should be stripped off if the growth has encroached upon it.

Hemorrhages from the choroidal vessel, if recent, appear in the fundus as round or oval spots of a brighter red than the surrounding tissues. If old, they are very apt to be mottled with black or white spots, and if the affected part of the choroid has become atrophic, a white spot, surrounded by a black border, may be present, the white appearance being due to the sclerotic and the black to heaping up of pigment. The only condition that resembles choroidal hemorrhages are those from the retinal vessels (see Disease of the Retina). The cause of choroidal extravasations are injuries to the eyeball, such as blows with blunt instruments, inflammation of the choriod, tears, etc. Hamamelis θ, a tablet three times a day, seems to hasten absorption of the blood.

Detachment of the choroid is a condition seldom diagnosed. It may be mistaken for a detached retina, from which it is to be distinguished by its smooth surface and absence of wave-like motion, and by its red color (see Detachment of the Retina); from a tumor by the tension of the eye remaining normal or sub-normal. If the tumor be vascular, that would be another diagnostic point. Treatment: none. Traumatic ruptures of the choroid generally are seen near the optic disk. The choroid may be torn near the ora serrata, but it is not possible to discover it during life. Immediately after the injury, the retina overlying the laceration becomes hazy. When this condition clears up, the rupture may be seen as a yellowish streak in the fundus, with extravasation of blood near its extreme edges. Later on, the tear becomes a pale, yellowish-white color, with more or less complete border of pigment. If the rupture is very small, it may look like a black line. The amount of impairment of vision depends upon the extent and location of the rupture. A very small tear involving the macula would cause a much greater disturbance than a very large one in a more peripheral part of the fundus. Treatment: keep the eyes at rest and protect them from bright light. Give Aconite 3x, a tablet every hour, if the patient is nervous and restless. Arnica 3x, if he complains simply of soreness of the eyeball. Nux vom. ix will be a good remedy in the later stages, to restore the function of the retina surrounding the injury, which seems to suffer more or less from shock.

Coloboma of the choroid is a defect of development, a segment of the lower or lower and inner part of the choroid being absent. The absence of the choroid at this place allows the white sclera to appear, and the retinal vessels may be seen passing over it, the pigment layer of the retina being also absent at this point. The so-called central coloboma is of doubtful origin.

Chapter Thirteen - Diseases of The Retina

Introduction.

The human retina, when normal and healthy, is transparent in all its parts, with the exception of its pigment layer and the blood that is circulating in its blood-vessels. The opacity of the pigment layer varies greatly. In persons of the blonde type it sometimes contains so little pigment that the larger choroidal vessels can be distinctly seen through it, so that the color of the fundus is a bright red. In very dark brunettes it is sufficiently opaque to give a very dark red tone to the fundus. In the negro and other dark races the tone of the fundus is a dark slate gray. When we speak of the ophthalmoscopic appearances of the healthy retinal vessels, we mean the red column contained in them, which is about one-third the diameter of the blood-vessel, the plasma and walls making up the other two-thirds. The cardinal objective symptoms of pathological changes of the retina are opacities and changes of contour, and of tint of the arteries and veins.

Opaque Optic Nerve Fibers

constitute an anomaly of the retina that might be mistaken for a pathological condition. They appear as white patches, generally near the optic disk, though not continuous with it. They extend for some distance from the disk, and may extend even beyond the macula lutea, around which they curve, but have never been observed to invade it. Their endings present a ravelled look, something like a flame. That the opacity is in the nerve fiber layer may be determined by the fact that it covers the retinal vessels.

The absence of all inflammatory or degenerative changes on the fundus distinguishes these opaque optic nerve fibers from diseased conditions. Being opaque, these fibers prevent the light from reaching the posterior layer of the retina; consequently that part of the eye occupied by them is blind. Post-mortem examinations have shown that the opacity of the fibers is due to the axis cylinder being covered by the myaline sheath, which ordinarily does not surround the fibers after they enter the eyeball. Without doubt the condition is congenital.

Hyperaemia of the Retina

may be active or passive. Active hyperaemia may be due to injury of the eye, or to eye-strain, or it may be the first stage of inflammation. It is diagnosed by the disk appearing redder than normal, and the vessels appearing larger and more torturous, the greatest change being in the veins. It is a condition not often recognized.

Passive hyperaemia is due to some obstruction to the return of blood. This obstruction may be systemic, or it may be caused by the pressure of a swollen optic nerve or a tumor in the orbit, or any extra-ocular trouble that interferes with the caliber of the retinal vessels, or it may be due to increased intra-ocular tension, as witnessed in Glaucoma. In this form the veins will be very much larger and more tortuous than the arteries, and the disk may be no redder than normal.

Anaemia of the Retina.

Simple anaemia is recognized by the small size and the straight course of the retinal vessels, and by the paleness of the optic disk.

RETINITIS.

Inflammation of the Retina.

Inflammation of the retina is commonly secondary to some constitutional disease. It has been frequently observed in the course of the following troubles: Bright's disease, diabetes, leucothemia, pernicious anaemia, oxaluria, syphilis, etc.

Retinitis Albuminuria.

The most striking picture of profound inflammation of the retina is the retinitis that is found in albuminuria; it may be present in any form of Bright's disease, or in the albuminuria of pregnancy, or in post-scarlatinal or diphtheritic nephritis. It is most frequently found with contracted kidney, and when accompanying this form of Bright's disease it is a bad symptom, the patient seldom living more than two years from the time the retinal changes take place. When found in pregnancy, scarlet fever, or diphtheria, the patients often recover with a fair amount of vision. Its appearance during pregnancy should be considered an indication of severe complication of kidney trouble, and always taken as a warning that the patient is in great danger. Sudden attacks of temporary blindness, even without retinal changes, should put the physician on guard, as they may be due to uremic poisoning. The term uremic amaurosis is applied to this condition.

Symptoms: The objective symptoms may consist of only a slight dimness of vision, or of any degree of poor sight, even of complete blindness, depending upon the location and stage of the disease. As a rule, there is no pain in the eyes. Distorted vision is a rare symptom, and, while retinitis is not the first symptom of Bright's disease, it is often the first one observed. The changes in the fundus, as seen with the aid of the ophthalmoscope, may be limited to a slight haze of the retina, and an indistinctness of the outlines of the optic disk and larger vessels. These are often the only objective symptoms in the primary stage of the disease. In some cases, in addition to these symptoms, numerous hemorrhages are to be seen scattered over the fundus, those in the nerve fiber being distinguished by their striated appearance. This striation is caused by the blood settling between the supporting fibers. Hemorrhages in the deeper parts of the retina have a mottled look, while those between the retina and vitreous look like red disks, the lower part of which is darker than the upper, due to the settling of the blood corpuscles, the serum of the blood occupying the upper part. These hemorrhages, in the early stage, before disintegration has set in, are of a brighter red than the rest of the fundus, and they may be found on any part of the retina or optic disk. The retinal vessels may be covered by, or run over, the hemorrhages. The hemorrhages may disintegrate and be absorbed without leaving any trace, or irregular masses of pigment may be seen during and after the absorption of the blood, or, as most commonly occurs, the blood undergoes fatty degeneration, the spots then becoming of a glistening white color, with the slightest tint of yellow. These spots may remain in the fundus for a long time, and finally be absorbed without leaving any trace. In other cases, they set up destructive changes in the retina and choroid, with resulting atrophic spots on their membranes. In still others, and what are considered the typical forms of albuminuric retinitis, the retinal veins are dilated and tortuous, sometimes to a very great degree, while the arteries are very narrow and run a very straight course.

Masses of white exudation, elevated above the plane of the surrounding retina, are seen about the optic disk. These masses often hide parts of the blood-vessels, which they cover and seem to surround; the masses often coalesce, forming a mound around the optic disk. In the region of the macula small spots of white exudation appear, arranged in such a manner that the macula looks like a white stellate figure with a red center — the fovea centralis. Hemorrhages of all sizes may be seen scattered over the fundus, some being so small that they can be seen only by direct ophthalmoscopy. The outlines of the vessels are lost, and seem to be surrounded by exudation. The parts of the retina not occupied by the white exudation look swollen, and partial detachment of the retina may take place. The optic disk may be swollen and its outlines lost; numerous hemorrhages may be seen scattered over its surface. When the optic disk becomes involved, the disease is called neuroretinitis. The objective symptoms may decrease during the course of the disease. In the later stages, when the exudation and hemorrhages have degenerated, the fundus may be covered with white spots, that glisten and sparkle; these are made up of fat and cholesterine. The vitreous nearly always remains clear in this trouble. Both eyes are generally attacked, though one may be affected some time before the other.

Pathology: The destructive changes are not limited to the retina. Postmortem examinations have shown the vessels of the choroid and the fibers of the optic nerve to be in a state of fatty degeneration. The first pathological change seems to be a low grade of inflammation, followed by fatty degeneration of the walls of the vessels, this condition of the vessels being in all probability the cause of the hemorrhages. The supporting tissue of the retina increases and undergoes fatty degeneration. The ganglionic cells become enlarged, the enlargement being a form of degeneration. The nerve fibers enlarge, and in their course are found roundish swellings, causing the fiber to look like a bipolar ganglionic cell; finally the fibers undergo fatty degeration and become atrophic. The hemorrhages cause a certain amount of mechanical destruction of the retinal elements, and the contraction of the fibrous tissue also tends to destroy the nerve tissue. The pigment layer seems to be but little affected. All the symptoms and ophthalmoscopic appearances given as occurring in albuminuria may occur in tumors of the brain, or in cases where no constitutional disease can be discovered. Under the last-mentioned condition the disease would be called idiopathic retinitis; but such cases are very rare, the author having seen but one such case.

Course and Progress: The course of this disease is very chronic, except in pregnancy when miscarriage takes place, and in scarlet fever and diphtheria. The prognosis is bad in the chronic forms of Bright's disease, and fairly good when due to pregnancy, scarlet fever and diphtheria.

Treatment must be guided by the constitutional disease. If pregnancy be the cause, premature delivery is to be advised. The eyes should be protected from bright light by gray spectacles, the patient kept in a warm, dry, sunny room, the temperature of which should never be allowed to fall below seventy degrees. Frequent hot baths and systematic exercise should be ordered, the skin being well rubbed to promote excretion. The diet should be nourishing, but non-stimulating, no alcohol in any form being allowed. Plenty of pure water should be drank, but in small quantities. Merc. corr. 3x, a tablet three times a day, has seemed to me to be the remedy most frequently indicated.

Diabetic Retinitis.

This occurs in the grave forms of diabetes, and generally in their later stages. It is a very rare disease compared to diabetic cataract, which is quite common. As a rule, the retinitis is of a lower grade than that of albuminuria, to which it bears a close resemblance, both in the character of the inflammatory exudations and hemorrhages. In most cases the changes around the macula are not so marked, while the hemorrhages are more profuse. Still the difference in the appearance of the retinal changes is not sufficiently distinctive to enable us to distinguish one disease from the other by the ophthalmoscopic appearances alone. The presence of sugar or albumen in the urine establishes the diagnosis. The pathological changes in the retina seem to be almost identical in the two diseases. I can give no reliable indication for the prescription of remedies, as the only cases of this form of retinitis that I have seen were so near death that but little chance was given to try the effects of medicines.

Leuksemic Retinitis

is a rare disease in this country. In it the blood in the retinal vessels becomes a pale orange color, and the whole fundus being more or less of this shade. The other symptoms are such as may be seen in the mild forms of albuminuric retinitis. In the treatment, consult Thuja and Natrum sulph.

Retinitis has been observed in pernicious oxaluria, liver disease, etc. There is nothing distinctive, ophthalmoscopically, about these forms, and the treatment will be that of general disease, together with protection of the inflamed retina by rest and dark glasses, as given under retinitis albuminuria.

Syphilitic Retinitis (see Syphylitic Choroido-retinitis).

Proliferating Retinitis.

In this form membranes form in the vitreous, which are seen to contain new vessels that are apparently connected with the retinal vessel. The cause of this trouble is uncertain; some writers think that the disease results from hemorrhage into the vitreous. Kali iod. or Thuja may be tried.

Retinitis Punctata Albescens

is a mild form of circumscribed retinitis, in which a number of small white spots are found in the retina between the optic disk and the macula. It is very apt to produce a central scotoma when it involves the macula. There may be some enlargement of the retinal veins and a few hemorrhages. The disease is quite rare, and its pathology not well understood. The indications for treatment will have to be obtained from the general system. Consult Merc, corr., Kali iod., Merc, biniod., Sulphur, Bell., etc.

Affections of the Retinal Vessels.

Embolism of the central artery of the retina.
Hemorrhage into the sheath of the optic nerve.
Thrombosis of the retinal vessels.
Spasm of the retinal arteries.
Hemorrhagic retinitis.
Apoplexy of the retina.
Perivasculitis.
Sclerosis of the retinal vessels.
Aneurisms and calcareous degeneration of the retinal vessels.

Embolism of the central artery presents one characteristic symptom — sudden blindness, generally limited to one eye. The objective symptoms that complete the diagnosis are great diminution in the size of the arteries; they sometimes appear as red and white threads, the red color being due to the blood corpuscles that have stagnated in the vessels. If the patient is seen immediately after the attack, these are all the changes that will be present. Later a faint grayish haze will have spread over the retina, out of which the fovea centralis will shine as a cherry-red spot, the bright color of the fovea being due to the contrast of the surrounding oedematous parts of the retina. Other reasons for this marked contrast are that there are no branches of the retinal artery in the fovea, that the retina is very thin at this point and the part of the choroid it covers very vascular. At this time the veins of the retina may look larger than normal, and present dilatations and contractions in their course. The blood having ceased to circulate, parts of the vein will appear congested and the other parts quite empty, depending upon the way they are affected by the intra-ocular tension. Later on, the vessels — both arteries and veins — atrophy and become the merest threads, the inner layer of the retina becomes white and atrophic, the eye being absolutely blind, though the layer of rods and cones may be apparently normal for years after the destruction of the retinal circulation The cause of all these changes is the plugging of the central artery by a fibrinous shred, which is generally derived from a diseased heart. If the embolic matter becomes septic, we no longer have the phenomenon of embolism, but that of septic retinitis. The embolism may affect only one branch of the retinal artery; then the changes described above are limited to a section of the retina, causing a gap in the visual field. All methods of treatment have so far failed. The retinal arteries being end arteries, there is no way in which a collateral circulation can be established. If the embolism has not entered the central artery, but only obstructs its orifice, where it is given off from the ophthalmic artery, it may be swept away, and then the circulation of the retina will be re-established; and if this occurs before the retina has become atrophic, sight may be restored. Hemorrhage into the sheath of the optic nerve may produce all the symptoms of embolism.

Thrombosis.

Thrombosis of the central vein is very difficult to distinguish from embolism of the artery. Hemorrhages of the retina are sometimes seen in embolism, though very rarely, while in thrombosis they are common and the retinal veins are apt to be engorged and tortuous. Loss of vision is not so complete or sudden as in embolism, though transient attacks of blindness often precede the ophthalmoscopic appearances. The prognosis should be guarded, as the disease is a very grave one, for the cerebral vessels may be in the same condition. Hamamelis might be a remedy.

Spasm of the Retinal Arteries.

This is a functional trouble. The symptoms are dimness of vision, with contraction of the vessels, the optic disk being very pale, bearing a close resemblance to atrophy. Poisoning by quinine is a frequent cause. Disturbances of the sympathetic nervous system are also frequent causes. It is to be distinguished from the atrophic form of retinitis by the absence of all other symptoms of that condition (see Atrophy of the Optic Nerve).

Nux vom. ix is the remedy; given three times a day, it will generally restore the function of the retina in a very short time.

Apoplexy of the Retina.

When there are hemorrhages into the retina without known cause — without symptoms of inflammation of the retina or nerve — the condition is termed apoplexy of the retina. The condition may be the forerunner of cerebral apoplexy. When haziness or other symptoms of retinitis appear, the disease is called hemorrhagic retinitis. Retinal hemorrhage, besides being a symptom of many forms of retinitis, may be due to traumatism, atheromatous degeneration of the vessels, glaucoma, scurvy, menstrual disturbances, etc. The injury to sight caused by retinal hemorrhages will depend upon their location and extent, the nearer the macula the more marked will be the symptoms and the less will be the hope of restoration of vision. Those that spread out between the retina and vitreous are less apt to do lasting harm than those that invade the deep tissues of the retina. Traumatic hemorrhages are generally more rapidly absorbed, and are less apt to undergo fatty degeneration, than those of the other forms. Next to these in rapidity of absorption come the hemorrhages due to menstrual disturbances. Those that are due to vascular disease are generally very slow of absorption, and are very certain to undergo fatty degeneration (see Hemorrhages in Albuminuria).

Treatment: The eyes should be protected from bright light, and the patient should not be allowed to read or do any fine work. Where there are symptoms of retinitis, and in simple hemorrhages due to menstrual disturbances, Belladonna ix or 3x will be found to be an excellent remedy. Aconite 3x, or Arnica 3x, in the traumatic forms; Aconite if the injury is of recent date, Arnica if of several days' standing. Hamamelis in cases where the hemorrhages recur, especially if they are large and the retina is free from signs of inflammation and degeneration. Phosphorus 6x, when the hemorrhagic spots are small and very numerous, and where they show a tendency to degeneration, especially if there be a low grade of retinitis present. The prognosis must always be guarded; though many cases recover with good vision, the patients are always liable to have a macular hemorrhage which may destroy vision.

Perivasculitis

is a localized retinitis occurring in the tissue that surrounds the vessels. As a rule, it does not involve the veins to as great an extent as the arteries. The vessels, or the parts of them affected, look like white cords. They are enlarged, their walls being thickened, but their caliber is not encroached upon to any extent, as the blood circulates through them. Peripheral vision is first affected. Small hemorrhages are found, and the parts of the retina close to the vessels are hazy. The disease is slowly progressive. It being a very rare disease we have not had sufficient experience to furnish indications for treatment. Aneurism, Sclerosis and Calcareous Degenerations of the retinal arteries may occur.

Detachment of the Retina.

This is a comparatively common affection. Black spots that seem to float before the eye, distortion of objects seen in certain parts of the visual field, a diminution of light-sense, a loss of part or of the entire visual field, or even complete blindness, are among the objective symptoms. Preceding the detachment the patient will often notice black spots, flashes of fire and colored lights before the eye. The detachment seldom takes place in both eyes at the same time, and only one eye may be attacked. The detachment does not include the pigment layer, it remaining in contact with the choroid. With the ophthalmoscope the detached retina can be recognized by a change of color of the detached part; it nearly always appears of a greenish-gray color, though in some cases the retina and fluid behind it are transparent, then there is no change of retinal tint; the vessels upon it are of a darker shade, and appear to be smaller than the vessels of the attached portion. In a majority of cases the detached portion will have a wavelike motion when the eye is moved. If the detachment is far forward, it may be seen by oblique illumination. If the entire retina is detached it may be impossible to make out the details of the fundus, the only thing seen being a gray mass that seems to be close to the lens. In the great majority of detachments the vitreous will be found to be fluid, and to contain floating opacities. In simple detachment, the intra-ocular tension is diminished. When the detachment is due to tumor, and in rare cases where it is complicated with glaucoma, the tension will be increased. In slight traumatic detachment, the tension may be normal. Traumatic detachments in healthy eyes are very uncommon, unless the injury is sufficient to destroy the eye. Cyclitis is a frequent cause of detachment; secondary detachment, due to this cause, is but a stage in the destruction of the eye due to the primary disease. Detachment takes place suddenly, and the upper part of the retina is more apt to be affected first, and as the fluid behind the retina sinks downward, the detachment increases downward. It may be very small at first, and then extend so as to involve the entire retina. Sometimes tears of the retina may be seen; they are recognized by the red choroid showing very vividly, and sometimes the curled edge of the tear may be seen. The pathological changes that precede and cause detachment are in all probability situated in the vitreous; changes taking place in that body cause parts of it to shrink away from the retina, the space between the vitreous and retina being filled with a watery fluid. The continued traction of the shrinking vitreous, aided by the diminished tension of the eye, causes the retina to become detached; this may take place by the retina tearing and allowing the fluid to rush behind it. Or, in the cases where there has been no tear, the irritation of the membranes of the eye, due to the traction of the contracting vitreous, aided by the diminished volume of that body, may cause a sudden secretion of fluid behind the retina, and so detaching it. The prognosis is unfavorable in all cases, but more so when the eye is highly myopic. But some detachments do become re-attached, and remain so; others relapse and become worse than before. Cataract is often found in connection with detachment of the retina. Treatment: Have the patient put to bed and kept on his back, with the eye firmly bandaged, without pressure on the cornea. Gels, ix should be given four times a day. With this treatment I have seen several detachments become reattached, and some of them remain so after the lapse of several years.

Retinitis Pigmentosa.

Synonyms: Sclerosis of the Retina, Pigmented Degeneration of the Retina, Fibroid Degeneration of the Retina, Atrophy of the Retina. Sclerosis of the retina may appear in two forms of degeneration; one in which the infiltration of pigment is the marked objective symptom, and the other in which no pigmentary changes can be seen with the ophthalmoscope, though microscopic examination shows that pigment is present in the retina to an abnormal amount. The objective symptoms are a concentric narrowing of the field of vision, with a marked torpor of the retina, while the patient's central vision may remain normal and his field of vision be of a fair extent when the objects are brightly illuminated. A slight reduction in the amount of light will cause a great diminution in the visual acuity of the central part of the retina, and a marked narrowing of the visual field. The peripheral parts of the retina seem to be affected more by reduced illumination than the central parts. Thus night blindness is so marked that a patient who can go about the crowded streets in the daytime becomes absolutely helpless in the evening, even if there be light enough to enable a person with normal eyes to see small objects distinctly. Sometimes the visual field becomes so small that the patient can only see straight ahead, even with good light, and in this case he could not walk about the streets with safety, even if the central vision equaled the normal.

Objective symptoms: The ophthalmoscopic picture in a typical fully developed case of retinitis pigmentosa is characteristic. In the early stages the only changes that can be seen may be an apparent narrowing of the retinal vessels; this appearance is due to a hyaline thickening of the vessel's walls, which does not increase the diameter of the vessels, but encroaches on its caliber, and so diminishes the diameter of the red blood stream. This degeneration of the vessels increases as the disease progresses, and the vessels look narrower, so that in time the smaller vessels may disappear from view. The optic disk loses its rosy tint of health, and becomes of a pale yellowish white. In the non-pigmented forms of sclerosis these may be the only changes visible with the ophthalmoscope. In the pigmented form lines of black pigment may be seen along the vessels, and delicate stellate lace-like figures between the forks of their branches, and sometimes parts of the arteries may be seen surrounded by a delicate network of pigment. The characteristic disposition of the pigment grannies is in the form of bone corpuscles, and these are generally found around the equator of the eye. With the progress of the disease they surround the macula more closely, but seldom encroach upon it, nor are they likely to involve the ora serrata. In the pure forms of retinitis pigmentosa there are no visible changes in the choroid, though certain parts of the fundus may look lighter than others, on account of the destruction of the pigment in the pigment layer. The disease that most closely resembles this degeneration of the retina is syphilitic choroido-retinitis. The latter disease will generally present some atrophic spots in the choroid, or some more or less rounded placque or ring-like deposits of pigment. The history will also assist in the differential diagnosis.

Etiology, Course and Prognosis: The cause of this trouble is unknown. The disease may be congenital, though the pigmentary changes seldom show early in life. Both eyes are usually attacked, though one may be further advanced than the other. This may serve as a diagnostic point between it and sclerosis, secondary to diseases of other parts of the eye. Its course is very slow, the patient sometimes reaching old age before the eyesight is completely destroyed, and there seem to be periods of remission, when the sight and field of vision will be improved. The slightest variation in the amount of light makes such a difference that mistakes are made unconsciously. The prognosis as to cure is bad, there being no case on record with restoration of the visual field. The secondary forms of pigmentary degeneration of the retina and choroid offer a much more favorable prognosis, and some of these may be easily mistaken for true retinitis pigmentosa and reported as cures.

Pathology: The pathological changes that have been described as taking place in this disease are primarily changes that cause an increase and subsequent contraction of the fibrous tissue, with a peculiar transparent thickening of the walls of the vessels. These changes lead to destruction of the nerve elements, partly by the pressure of the constricting tissue, and partly by diminished nutrition. As a natural consequence the peripheral parts of the retina will first suffer, because there is a much greater amount of connective tissue in the peripheral parts, and because the vessels of this part are smaller, and a very slight change in the vessels will greatly impede the flow of blood. Treatment so far has not been satisfactory. There are two remedies that suggest themselves, and should be tried in the absence of indications for other remedies — Nux vom. and Phos. In some cases in which I have used these drugs the patients have expressed themselves as seeming better, but no case has remained under my treatment for a sufficient number of years to determine whether there was any permanent improvement.

INJURIES OF THE RETINA.

Ruptures of the Retina — Burns of the Retina.

Blows on the eye sometimes cause impairment of vision, with only slight signs of oedema of the retina. This condition is called Conmotio-retinae. Ruptures of the retina may be the result of concussion of the eyeball by bodies moving with great velocity, such as corks from bottles containing effervescent fluids. Uncomplicated, traumatic tears of the retina are very rare. The diagnosis is made by the ophthalmoscope; the torn edges may be seen, and sometimes one or more of the retinal vessels may be found torn across.

Burns of the retina generally occur from looking at the sun with the unprotected eye. They may be very slight or severe, depending upon the length of time the eye was exposed to the glare. Looking for a length of time at a glowing furnace, or at an electric light, may produce the same results. The prognosis will depend upon the amount of injury; slight cases may recover very rapidly and completely, severe ones very slowly, and sometimes central vision is entirely destroyed.

Treatment: Protect the eyes by gray glasses, and do not allow the eyes to be used. Belladonna 3x will be found a useful remedy, given three times a day.

Tumors of the Retina.

Glioma is the only malignant growth that originates from the retinal tissue. It occurs iu children only. It causes the pupil to present a bright yellow or whitish reflex. The only condition that glioma is liable to be mistaken for is localized septic choroiditis, and from that it can be distinguished by the history of inflammatory symptoms, and perhaps the remains of past inflammation of the iris or choroid. In the early stages of glioma there are no inflammatory symptoms nor increase of tension. Later the eye becomes very hard, and the eyeball very red and painful; the growth may burst the eyeball, or it may extend to the brain along the course of the optic nerve. After the eyeball has ruptured the contents of the orbit may become a fungous mass. The lymphatic glands and liver may be secondarily implicated. Death may result either by extension to the brain, or by implication of other vital organs, or from general exhaustion. The only treatment is removal of the eye at once. If the optic nerve or orbit has become involved there is very little hope of prolonging life; while a prompt removal, when the disease is still confined to the retina, will, in all probability, put an end to the trouble.

Cystoid Degeneration of the Retina.

This is a rare condition that has been discovered post-mortem. Daring life a retinal tumor would, in all probability, be mistaken for a detachment of the retina.

Cysticerci may be retinal, giving rise to what appears to be detachment of that membrane.

Hyperaemia of the Optic Nerve.

This condition is considered to be present when the optic disk is redder than normal. There is such variation in the tint of normal optic disks that it is frequently very difficult, when the hyperaemia is not great, to say that it does exist. If only one eye be affected, it will greatly aid the diagnosis by comparing it with the unaffected eye. Hyperaemia of the disk may be a symptom of Neuritis, Retinitis, Choroiditis, Cyclitis, Iritis, etc.

It may also be present in refractive defects. When the vitreous is hazy, the disk will appear redder than it really is. The treatment of hyperaemia, when it is not a part of an inflammatory condition of other parts of the eye, is to correct any refractive defect that may exist, to rest the eyes, and protect them from strong light.

Belladonna 3x, a tablet three times a day, will be found of great value in relieving the condition.

Diseases of the Optic Nerve.

Choked disk, oedema of the optic papilla, choked neuritis, papillitis, neuritis, descending neuritis, axial neuritis. Of these terms, the first two should be limited to diseases of the optic papilla, in which the only symptom is an oedematous swelling of the intra-ocular portion of the optic nerve, with swelling and tortuosity of the retinal veins.

Choked neuritis and papillitis express a form of optic neuritis, limited to the part of the nerve contained in the lamina cribrosa and the eyeball, in which the oedema and swelling of the papillae and tortuosity and swelling of the retinal veins are marked, while the inflammatory changes are slight, consisting of opacities of the disk, with more or less hemorrhagic exudations. The outline of the disk is not lost nor is the retina involved.

Neuritis, descending neuritis and neuro-retinitis are the terms used when the inflammatory changes are the marked symptoms. The disk will have lost its transparency, and will be either red, gray, or white, or mottled with all these colors. Hemorrhages may be scattered over it, or over the adjoining retina. The disk will be swollen, sometimes markedly so, and its outline lost in the retina, this latter structure being nearly always affected. The swelling and tortuosity of the veins are well marked, though they are never engaged to the extent found in choked disk or choked retinitis. The exudation and swelling of the papillae often bury portions of the retinal vessels. The form of neuritis described above is not limited to the intraocular part of the nerve, but involves its continuity. It is for this reason that the term neuritis is applied to it.

Retro-bulbar neuritis and axial neuritis are conditions that present no characteristic ophthalmoscopic symptoms during the active stage of the disease.

While, in some cases, it is very easy to distinguish the various forms of choked disk and neuritis, in others it is impossible, owing to one form merging into another, and from the fact that the causes of any of these troubles may be located within the cranium, or due to constitutional diseases. The treatment of the various forms is very similar. For these reasons we will treat all the affections of the intra-ocular part of the optic nerve under one head, making distinctions only where it seems to be absolutely necessary to a proper understanding of the subject.

Retro-bulbar and axial neuritis will be treated together.

Symptoms: There may be no subjective symptoms in choked disk or choked neuritis, and even in neuritis and neuro-retinitis the subjective symptoms may be limited to a slight haziness of objects. On the other hand, sight may be completely lost very early in the disease. A peculiarity of these troubles is that the intensity of the pathological changes in the nerve, as revealed by the ophthalmoscope, may not correspond with the state of the vision. In some cases, where there are few, if any, objective symptoms, the patient may be blind, while in others, where the objective symptoms are marked, there may be little or no impairment of vision. But as a rule, the impairment of sight is greater in neuro-retinitis than in choked disk or choked neuritis. Headache, dizziness, loss of memory, or other symptoms that do not seem in any way related to the eye, may bring the patient to consult you.

Objective symptoms will be ophthalmoscopic, and limited to the optic disk and retina, the refractive media not being affected. In simple oedema, or choked disk, the optic papilla will project into the vitreous to the extent of several mm., the retinal arteries will be small, and the retinal veins will be larger and very tortuous. The swollen tissue may present a translucent, grayish look; although the disk is so greatly swollen, its outline is not lost. The above-described conditions may be only the early stage of choked neuritis, or they may constitute the entire trouble. In choked neuritis, reddish spots due to hemorrhage, and opaque masses due to exudation and proliferation of cellular elements and to changes in the nerve fibers of an inflammatory character, will be seen.

In descending neuritis or neuro-retinitis the papilla will look red and inflamed, the small vessels on it being very prominent, while the retinal veins will not be engaged to the extent found in choked disk or choked neuritis. The arteries may be but slightly enlarged or even smaller and straighter than normal. The tissue of the disk may be gray or white, or it may be mottled with gray, white, and red. The disk may be very slightly or greatly swollen, its outlines will be lost, the surrounding retina participating in the inflammation. The macula lutea may be occupied by whitish masses arranged in a stellate form, similar to the condition found in retinitis albuminuria. Hemorrhages in the papilla and surrounding retina are common. The vessels will often be covered in their course by inflammatory exudation. Atrophic changes in the disk may appear as late symptoms in any of the forms of choked disk or neuritis given above.

Etiology and Pathology: The cause of choked disk and choked neuritis is, as a rule, some intra-cranial trouble, which causes an increase in the intra-cranial tension. Such tension or pressure interferes with the circulation of the intra-ocular lymph, and also causes distension of the sheaths of the optic nerve near the eyeball, where the sheaths are weakest, resulting in an ampullary dilatation. As a consequence of these conditions, the tissue of the lamina cribrosa swells and constricts the nerve fibers and retinal vessels, and the disk becomes swollen. The pressure may be so great or so long continued that atrophy of the nerve fibers results, without any antecedent inflammation, or, the cause being removed before atrophic changes have taken place, the nerve will become functionally and structurally normal.

Inflammatory changes may be added, either as a result of the pressure interfering with the nutrition of the disk sufficiently to cause disintegration of some tissue, the products of which will be sufficiently irritating to set up inflammatory changes in other parts of the disk, or the fluid that is poured out of the brain may be sufficiently irritating to inflame the choked and naked axis cylinder of the optic disk. A frequent cause is tumors of the brain, especially those located in the posterior portion, tumors of the spinal cord, and grave constitutional diseases, such as albuminuria and diabetes, or it may result from great loss of blood, hydrocephalus, etc.

Both eyes are generally affected, though, even when the cause is a cranial tumor, only one eye may be involved, on account of proliferation of the fixed and exuded cells resulting in the formation of new fibrous tissue, which contracts and destroys the nerve fibers by pressure. The number of nerve fibers is less, and the amount of connective tissue greater, in the part of the nerve that has been affected. This will make the disk appear whiter and larger. Extravasation, with a subsequent fatty degeneration of the exuded blood, may occur. The causes of descending neuritis are such as set up inflammatory changes within the cranium, meningitis being probably the most frequent. Both eyes are generally affected; though, even when the cause is a cranial tumor, only one eye may be involved. In children, no doubt, many of the atrophic changes seen in the optic nerve are due to meningitis. Diseases of the orbit and facial erysipelas are also causes, and in such cases only one eye may be affected. In descending neuritis, the inflammation extends from the cranial cavity by continuity of tissue, either the interstitial tissue or the sheaths of the nerve being the medium. The formation and contraction of new cicatricial tissue may involve the entire nerve, or only some of its fibers; upon the extent of these changes will depend the amount of vision remaining after the disease subsides.

Course and Prognosis: The course and prognosis of choked disk, choked neuritis, and descending neuritis are dependent upon the affection that causes them. Such causes as syphilitic tumors, simple meningitis, erysipelas, and diseases of the orbit offer the most favorable prognosis. In cases caused by malignant growths and tubercular meningitis, the prognosis is bad. In all cases the prognosis should be guarded, as the neuritis is often a very late symptom of inter-cranial trouble, the patient dying before the disease of the papilla has reached its height. The general symptoms must guide in predicting the course of the disease of the nerve. Though all forms of intra-ocular neuritis run a slow course, some may be cured in a few weeks, while others will require months. Recovery may take place with complete restoration of vision, or with impaired vision, or a contracted visual field, or blindness may result.

Treatment: The patient should be confined to the house, or even to his bed, depending upon his general condition. His eyes should be protected from bright light by gray glasses, and he should be treated as a very sick person, remembering that the eye trouble may be only a symptom of a fatal disease. If a syphilitic history is obtained, or the patient presents symptoms of this disease, the treatment should be that of constitutional syphilis. In the non-syphilitic cases the remedies which have given ine the best results are

Gels. θ, or Bry. θ, in simple choked disk, and Hellebor. when the case is one of choked neuritis. Puls. θ, Bell, θ or Veratrum vir. θ are the remedies to be studied. In descending neuritis also Merc. corr. 3x, Cuprum met. 3x, and Arsenicum 33c It is impossible to give indications limited to the eyes in this disease, as they are in nowise characteristic. The disease being secondary, the symptoms must be derived from the general system. If the patient be suffering from syphilis — and this is one of the most frequent causes — it is best to give him large doses of Kali iod., for the purpose of causing destruction and absorption of the growth, which we may assume is the cause of the neuritis. After this absorption has been accomplished, as evidenced by the disappearance of the neuritis, the patient should be treated by giving him the indicated remedies. The iodide of potash will not, in my opinion, cure the neuritis, but it is a most valuable agent to destroy syphilitic growths, which, if not promptly destroyed, might cause death by pressure on some vital part of the brain. Nux vom. θ, a tablet three times a day, will be found to be an excellent remedy after the inflammatory symptoms have subsided, vision being often greatly improved by its long-continued use, no matter what the cause of the neuritis may have been.

Retro-bulbar Neuritis, Axial Neuritis.

As these forms present no characteristic ophthalmoscopic symptoms, we must depend upon other methods of examination to establish diagnosis, and among these the art of measuring the visual field is the most important. Rough measurement may be made by placing the patient opposite the examiner, about two feet distant, and having him look directly at the examiner's finger, which should be held directly in front of the patient's eye, and about twelve inches from it; then the examiner should use the index finger of his other hand, bringing it into view first from above, noting the greatest distance from the fixed finger at which it is seen, and so on around the circle. The examiner decides whether there is any contraction of the visual field by comparison with his own. To make anything like an accurate examination, some form of perimeter will be required. The ordinary perimeter is a metal band, in the shape of a half circle, supported by a stand with a suitable chinrest, so placed that the patient's eye is at the distance of the radius of curvature of the half circle, which rotates about a center containing the fixation point for the patient. A disk which is graduated in degrees is attached to the stand behind the half circle; by this arrangement the position of the semicircular arm may be noted. The arm itself is also graduated in degrees, from zero to 90°, the fixation point being zero on the scale. A carriage containing a test object, generally a white or colored disk, moves freely on the arm. By sliding the carriage along the arm, and by rotating the arm around the circle, the visual field may be measured very well. Charts of concentric circles crossed by radii, both the circles and radii being numbered in degrees, are prepared to correspond with the markings on the perimeter. To examine and record the field of vision, the arm of the perimeter is placed in the vertical position, which is marked zero. The eye under examination is directed to the fixation point. The carriage containing the test disk is placed at the extreme upper end of the perimeter arm, then moved slowly along towards the fixation point. As soon as the patient sees the disk he should indicate the fact. The examiner should impress him with the importance of keeping his eye fixed upon the fixation point. Ask him if he sees two disks at the same time; if he does, then the place on the arm and the position of the arm should be marked on the chart by placing a cross on the circle and radius corresponding with parts of the perimeter indicated by them. The whole field should be gone over in this way, by rotating the arm and moving the disk. After the field has been taken in this way, then the disk should be placed at the fixation point, and moved towards the end of the arm, and so on throughout the field; the two charts should then be compared. The normal visual field varies in extent in its different parts. The upper part of the field will, on an average, equal 45 , the lower one 70 , the outer one 90 , and the inner one from 55 to 60°, the height of the nose influencing it. Priestly Smith's suggestion to record the visual field along radii separated by 45 ° is a good one, in the absence of a recording chart. The normal fields of the right and left eye would appear as follows:

This division would indicate the condition of the field, sufficiently accurate for all practical purposes. The measurements here given are only applicable when the test object is about 15 mm. in diameter, and of a white color. If a smaller or colored object is used the field would be smaller, and the different colors have different fields; red and green fields, as a rule, are smaller than those of blue and yellow. The amount and kind of light will also influence the field. Within the visual field, when the eye is normal, there should be no gaps, except the blind spot caused by the optic disk. In a field taken at one foot distant, the blind spot would be about 25 mm. in diameter, and it would appear to the outer side, and a little below the fixation point. To test for scotoma, near the central part of the visual field, a very large blackboard is best; one of about two meters will answer, the patient being placed two mm. from it and directed to fix a small chalk mark in the center of the board. Small pieces of paper are used, varying in diameter from one to ten millimeters, depending upon the fineness of the test required. The papers are made of different colors, so as to test for color scotoma. The test objects are placed on the ends of long black rods, and moved over the field, the outline of the blind spots being marked on the board. It is to be remembered that all defects are greatly magnified when the field is taken at this distance, compared with a field taken at the ordinary distance.

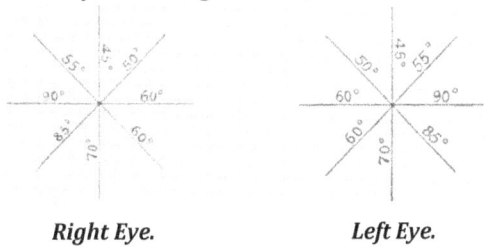

Right Eye.   *Left Eye.*

Retro-bulbar neuritis and axial neuritis may be acute or chronic, and may affect any part of the optic nerve. In many cases only the papillo-macular fibers are affected, in which case the disease is called axial neuritis. Acute retro-bulbar neuritis is characterized by sudden impairment of vision, without ophthalmoscopic changes to account for it. When the inflammation is localized close to the eyeballs there may be some hyperaemia of the disk and enlargement of the retinal veins. Sometimes there is pain when the eye is moved or pressed into the orbit. At other times the only symptom is loss of vision, which may vary from a slight haziness to complete blindness. If only the central fibers are affected, a central scotoma for colors may be present, red and green being the colors most frequently lost in the earlier stages; later on, all color sense may disappear from the central field, or even the light sense may be lost. The disease may terminate in recovery, or in complete or partial atrophy of the optic nerve. If only the central fibers have been affected, the atrophy may be confined to the outer third of the optic disk, taking the form of a sector, the apex of which is directed to the center and the base to the temporal side of the disk. The pathogenesis of retro-bulbar neuritis is obscure, on account of the absence of characteristic symptoms. If the patient recovers with good sight, we can never be certain that there has been an inflammation of the optic nerve. If atrophy of the disk results, even that may not be due to an inflammation of the nerve; the trouble may have been in the brain or spinal cord. Post-mortem examinations show that there are such diseases of the optic nerve as retrobulbar and axial neuritis. For these reasons we will treat the diseases in which the retro-bulbar part of the nerve is affected under the head of functional troubles.

Amblyopia — this term will be used to express conditions of poor sight, where the cause of the impairment cannot be assigned with any degree of certaintv.

Toxic amblyopia — chronic poisoning by tobacco, alcohol, bisulphide of carbon, stramonium, etc. — may be associated with visual disturbances, which have a close resemblance to the symptoms of chronic axial neuritis. Whether this is the pathological condition in the amblyopia due to these causes (if they are causes), or if the lesion is in the brain, are disputed points, there not having been sufficient number of post-mortem examinations made to determine. The great majority of cases recover with more or less perfect vision.

Symptoms: In tobacco amblyopia, which has been more thoroughly studied than the other forms, the characteristic symptom is a scotoma for red, in the part of the visual field corresponding to the part of the retina extending from the optic nerve to the outer side. The defect in the visual field will be of an oval shape; in the very slight form there may be only a tendency to confuse red and its complementary color, green, or the color may only look a little dim. In other cases, there may be a tendency to confuse blue and yellow> or the scotoma may be complete, so that this part of the eye may be blind. There is only one other symptom which is found in a great many cases — *i.e.*, the confusion of vision due to bright light, the patient asserting that he can see much better in a subdued light, and sometimes they really seem to do so. Tobacco amblyopia is found generally after the fortieth year, in men who are debilitated and in a general depressed condition, though it is sometimes found in young, strong and apparently vigorous men. It has also beeu found in women. The patients presenting this trouble may have used great quantities of tobacco for years before the first symptom appeared, or they may have been very moderate smokers, or they may have been chronic drunkards, who used large amounts of tobacco. In my own experience, I have never seen a case of amblyopia that I could attribute to the use of tobacco alone. In all cases of which I have any recollection the patients were addicted to both alcohol and tobacco. This group of troubles can not be distinguished from each other with any degree of certainty, and the treatment of them all is the same. Remove the supposed cause. Insist that the patient give up at once the use of tobacco and alcohol, or whatever seems to be the exciting cause. Advise an out-of-door life, and give Nux vom. 1x, a tablet three times a day. As a rule, the prognosis is good, if treatment has begun early. Be on your guard in all these obscure forms of trouble, as some such cases may not be due to these causes, and may result in blindness. There are other forms of defective sight without apparent lesion, such as congenital amblyopia, amblyopia ex anopsia, scintillating scotoma, hysterical amblyopia, etc., that are worthy of study, but lack of space forbids our making more than a mere mention of them. The examination of the eyes of young children, especially the children of the poor, will show that a certain number have not the normal acuteness of vision, and that the most careful correction of any refractive error from which they may be suffering will not make their vision perfect. When nothing can be found to account for the condition, it is called congenital amblyopia. In my experience, the early correction of refractive errors, if any exist, will greatly improve the vision if the patient wears the glasses all the time except when asleep.

Scintillating scotoma is, in all probability, due to some disturbance of the cerebral circulation. It may be a symptom of sick headache — the so-called blind headache — again, it may be a symptom of no importance, or it may be an early symptom of some serious nervous trouble. Hysterical amblyopia may assume all sorts of forms. The field of vision may be contracted, the central vision may be lost, color sense may be impaired or increased, the vision may be very good and fail suddenly during the examination and then become very good again, or there may be complete blindness for several days or weeks, followed by sudden restoration of sight, or the trouble may assume the form of the non-inflammatory diseases of the eye. The diagnosis will have to be made by the history of the case and the general symptoms. The remedy that I have found to be of greatest value is Zinc. val. 1x, a tablet every two hours.

Color-Blindness.

The color-blind may be divided into two classes, the first including those in whom the defect is congenital, and the second, those in which some disease of the eye or brain is the cause. The second class has been described under the head of acquired color-blindness, description of which will be found under the head of various diseases that cause this condition. The congenital form, from a practical standpoint, may be divided into two classes; the first, in which the color sense seems to be simply blunted, in which the patient requires a good light and an unusual amount of time to distinguish complementary colors and their shades and tints, especially if the atmosphere is at all hazy. The second class includes two degrees — the first, by far the most common, in which the patient fails to distinguish between green and red, these appearing to him as different tints of the same color. In this class will be found some patients who fail to distinguish between blue and yellow. This is very rare. To make a scientific examination and classification of color-blindness requires much study, thought, and time, and costly instruments, a description of which would not be suitable in an elementary work. Two tests, one known as Oliver's worsted test, and the other as the lantern test, are all that the practical examiner will require. The material for Oliver's test, consists of one skein each of green, red, rose, blue and yellow worsted. These colors should be pure, and the skeins of a larger size than the skeins which are to be matched with them. The match skeins are five in number, and are tints of the colors of the test skeins. In addition to these are eighteen other skeins, the colors of which are formed by a mixture of two or more of the colors of the test skeins. To simplify the recording of the test, attach to each skein a tag indicating the color and saturation. To make the examination, throw the skeins upon a black surface and select from the lot one of the test skeins, by preference the green, and give it to the patient, requesting him to select the three nearest matches, and place them by the test skein in their order of resemblance. The same procedure should be gone through with all the test skeins, and the result noted. The kind of mistakes made will indicate the kind and degree of color-blindness. The patient must not be asked to name the colors, as the mistakes in naming might only indicate color ignorance and not colorblindness. The lantern test is made when the examiner wishes to demonstrate that the candidate's perception and knowledge of color is not sufficient to warrant his occupying a position where the ability to recognize signals, quickly and accurately in all kinds of weather, is essential to the safety of life and property. The lantern is one in which the light is covered by an opaque hood, containing an opening, in front of which colored opaque glasses may be placed. The glasses used are a standard red and green, and several varieties of ground, ribbed, and fluted slides. The lantern should be at least fifteen feet from the candidate, the red and green glasses placed alternately in the opening, and the gray and other glasses placed over the colored one, in order to produce the effect of fog, mist, snow, rain and other atmospheric disturbances, under which conditions the various signals may have to be recognized. The person examined should be required to promptly name the colors as they appear. Care must be taken that he does not see the changes being made. In testing the colorvision only one eye should be examined at a time. So far no practical remedy has been discovered for the relief of congenital color-blindness. Both the worsted and lantern test apparatus may be obtained from dealers.

Chapter Fourteen - Glaucoma

This disease is characterized by a hardening of the eyeball and an excavation of the optic disk, although at the time of the examination only one of these symptoms may be present. Other symptoms, any or all of which may be found, are a prismatic-colored ring around the source of artificial light. This ring is some distance from the flame, and by that fact it is distinguished from the ring that is due to errors of refraction, the latter being close to the flame. Pain which takes the form of a ciliary neuralgia, the side of the face and head being involved. This pain may be very slight, the patient complaining of only a dull headache, or it may be of such severity as to cause vomiting and delirium, simulating an attack of meningitis. Haziness and loss of the normal sensitiveness of the cornea, touch giving no pain or reflex action. Dilatation of the anterior ciliary veins. Hyperaemia of the ocular and palpebral conjunctiva and swelling of the lids; shallowing of the anterior chamber; dilatation and immovability of the pupil; a greenish reflex from the eye — this latter symptom gave the disease its present name of glaucoma. Loss of vision and contraction of the visual field, which, as a rule, is more marked on the nasal side; arterial pulsation on the disk and flashes of fire before the eyes. Glaucoma is classified as primary when it occurs in an otherwise healthy eye; secondary when, it is the result of another disease. Primary glaucoma is classified into simple and inflammatory. Simple glaucoma, or glaucoma simplex, is a type in which there are no inflammatory symptoms. Progressive loss of sight, with contraction of the visual field, may be the only symptom complained of; objective examination may or may not show an increased hardness of the eyeball. To determine the tension of the eyeball, the patient should be directed to look downward, while gentle pressure is made upon the upper part of the eyeball (above the cornea), through the eyelids, with the index fingers of both hands alternately. The amount of resistance offered by the eyeball will indicate the tension of the eye, estimated by comparing it with a healthy eye of the same age. The younger the eye the less resistance does it offer, as a rule. The ability to estimate the degree of intra-ocular tension, with any degree of precision, can only be acquired by considerable practice, and for this reason the physician should make it a rule to note the tension of every eye he examines. The sign Tn is used to denote normal tension, and — T and + T denote, respectively, decrease and increase of tension, while — T, + Ti, — T2 and + T3 indicate degrees of increase of tension, varying from a very slight degree to stony hardness.

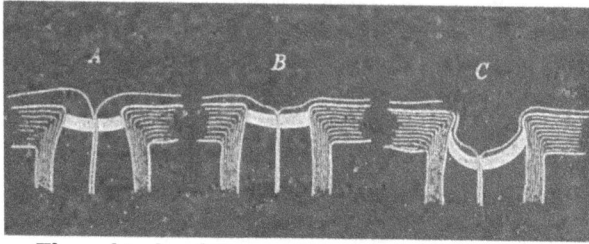

Three kinds of excavations of the optic nerve:
(a) Physiological Excavations,
(b) Atrophic Excavations.
(c) Glaucomatous Excavations.

The objective symptom most constant is an excavation of the optic disk, due to a yielding of the lamina cribrosa to the intra-ocular tension, and an atrophy of the optic nerve fibers. There are three kinds of excavation of the intra-ocular end of the optic nerve. The physiological occupies only apart of the disk, is funnel-shaped, and is due to nerve fibers separating at some distance below the plane of the retina before curving over to form it. It appears as a funnel-shaped depression, near the center of the disk, of a whiter color than the rest of the optic papilla. The atrophic excavation is shallow, and generally occupies the entire surface of the disk, and is of a whiter color, due to the fact that the nerve fibers have become atrophic and opaque. There can be no great depth to either the physiological or atrophic excavation, on account of the lamina cribrosa retaining its position. The glaucomatous excavation, like the atrophic, occupies the entire extent of the disk, and may be shallow or very deep; its edges may even overhang, depending upon the stage of the disease. If the affection be of recent date, and the excavation still shallow, the color of the disk will be normal; if of long standing, and the excavation deep, it may be very white or bluish, due to a secondary atrophy of the disk, the bluish shade being due to the fibers of the lamina cribrosa becoming visible on account of the wasting nerve fibers. The retinal vessels will be found crowded to one side of the disk, and, if the excavation be deep, they will be seen to bend sharply over to the edge of the nerve. If the edge of the disk is overhanging, part of the vessels will appear to be lost in passing from nerve to retina. The depth of the excavation may be measured by direct ophthalmoscopy, as refraction is measured (see chapter on Refraction). In the indirect examination an idea of the depth of the excavation may be obtained by moving the object lens from side to side, when the bottom of the excavation will be seen to move under the edge, and the greater the difference in the amount of movement of these two parts of the fundus the greater is the depth of the excavation. In the case of some of the shallow excavations it is almost impossible to distinguish between an atrophic and a glaucomatous excavation. In such cases other symptoms must be relied upon to establish the diagnosis. If the tension be found increased, that would decide in favor of glancoma, and the tension should be taken repeatedly, at different times, as it may vary greatly, even during the day. Greater contraction of the visual field, with normal color sense, would favor a diagnosis of glaucoma. As a rule, there is very little pain in glaucoma simplex; it runs a chronic course; its duration, till the final destruction, may be from two to twenty years. At any stage it may take on the inflammatory form, and the sight may be destroyed in a few hours. Increased tension is, in all probability, the essential cause of the destructive changes in this disease, although, at the time of examination, no increase of tension may be present. Without doubt, if the examinations are made with sufficient frequency, an increase of tension will be found, as the history of these cases, with the final blindness and stony hardness of the eyeball, show them to belong to the glaucomatous group.

Inflammatory Glaucoma.

Glaucoma inflammatorium is distinguished from glaucoma simplex by the presence of hyperaemia and oedema of the conjunctiva, swelling of the eye-lids, and engorgement of the ciliary veins. This disease has been divided into three stages. The first, or prodromal stage, may last weeks, months or years; the symptoms are intermittent attacks of dimness of sight, with weakness of accommodation, halo around the light, a slight neuralgia or dull headache, a dilated and sluggish pupil. The anterior chamber will be shallower than normal, and the cornea hazy. There may be slight hyperaemia of the ciliary zone, and tension will be increased. These attacks may occur quite frequently, even every day; they are nearly always relieved by sleep and brought on by grief, mental worry, or anything that causes an engorgement of the venous system. What distinguishes this stage from the second or glaucoma evolutura is, that these symptoms pass away and leave the vision of the eye normal. An attack of acute glaucoma is the beginning of the second stage. In this all the symptoms of the prodromal stage appear intensified. The eyeball is much harder, the sight very dim, the field greatly contracted, the pupil widely dilated, very sluggish and sometimes discolored, owing to the hazy media and the dilatation; the cornea very hazy and non-sensitive to touch; the ciliary veins injected, the lids and conjuctiva hypersemic and often swollen. Ciliary neuralgia is often so severe as to cause vomiting. A drop of Atropine will often set up an acute attack in an eye predisposed to glaucoma; for this reason the eyes of all elderly persons should be carefully examined for glaucomatous symptoms before instilling a mydriatic. The conditions that precede the prodromal symptoms may also excite an acute attack of glaucoma. An ophthalmoscopic examination is generally impossible during an acute attack, on account of the hazy condition of the cornea and humors. As soon as the media clear up the fundus should be examined; pulsation of the retinal veins or arteries, or both, may be found. An excavation may also be found, its depth depending upon the length of time the disease has lasted; it is rarely found during the first attack of acute glaucoma, unless several subacute attacks have preceded it. This attack will pass away in a measure. The cornea will clear up. The sight will improve, but it will not become what it was before the attack. The tension will grow less, but will still remain above the normal. The pain and congestion will disappear, and the patient will think he is recovering, but after a longer or shorter interval this attack will be followed by another, and so on, each attack destroying some sight, until the eye becomes blind and of a stone-like hardness. This stage is termed the third, or glaucoma absolutum. In this stage the cornea is clear and bright, but anesthetic. The pupil is very large. The dilated anterior ciliary veins stand out very clearly on the bluish-white sclera. The optic disk will be found deeply excavated and atrophic. The final result is that of glaucomatous degeneration, during which the patient is annoyed by flashes of light and attacks of pain, which only cease when the eyeball becomes shriveled, which may result by simple atrophy of the eyeball, or abscess of the cornea, or iridocyclitis may set in; or panophthalmitis, followed by phthsis bulbi, may be the final result.

Glaucoma fulminans is the term given to an attack of glaucoma of such severity that it destroys the sight in a few hours.

Chronic glaucoma runs a slow course, the first stage merging into the second. The symptoms are the same as in acute glaucoma, but modified. Though more slowly, the sight is no less surely destroyed than in the other forms of glaucoma.

Inflammatory glaucoma attacks both eyes, though there may be an interval of years between the attacks. It occurs, as a rule, between the fiftieth and seventieth years. It is more frequent among women than among men. Hyperopic eves seem more predisposed to this trouble; in fact, highly myopic eyes are seldom if ever attacked.

Glaucoma simplex is often found among the young and myopic; no age or refractive state of the eye is exempt.

Pathology: The pathology of glaucoma is obscure. The cause is a disturbance between the secretion and excretion of the humors of the eye. Anatomical examinations sometimes show a blocking up of the filtration spaces of the anterior chamber, though sometimes no such changes are found. The theories regarding the causes of the increase of tension are many and contradictory, and we do not feel warranted in discussing them.

Treatment: The only treatment that has been proven to be worthy of reliance in arresting this disease is an iridectomy, which should be large, the incision for which should be made in the sclera.

(For technique of iridectomy see chapter on Operations.)

The instillation of a solution of Eserine (1 to 200) to contract the pupil may be used with advantage pending an iridectomy. Eserine, in common with other myotics, has the property of reducing intra-ocular tension; unfortunately it cannot be continued indefinitely.

Atropine should not be used, as dilatation of the pupil by this drug will often precipitate an attack of glaucoma in an eye predisposed to this disease. We know of no medicine that can be depended upon to arrest an attack of glaucoma. Bryonia θ will often relieve the pain. Iridectomy is of greatest value in acute inflammatory glaucoma, and of least value in glaucoma simplex of long standing. Nevertheless, this operation should be made in in all forms of glaucoma and in any stage, as the eye is certain to be lost without it. In secondary glaucoma, more especially in the hemorrhagic form, the results of iridectomy are apt to be bad, the escape of the aqueous humor and consequent sudden reduction of tension resulting in hemorrhage from the intra-ocular vessels.

Buphthalmus, or Congenital Glaucoma.

As a result of increase of tension, during intra-uterine life the eye becomes enlarged in all its diameters. The cornea is larger than normal and the anterior chamber deeper. In this respect it differs from an adult glaucomatous eye, in which the anterior chamber is more shallow than normal. The course of the disease also diners, as spontaneous arrest of the disease sometimes occurs in the congenital form. The thinness and weakness of the cornea and sclera in the undeveloped eye allows the eye to become enlarged in all its diameters. The disease is rare, and no treatment has as yet been found to be of any value in restoring the eye.

Diseases with Diminution of Intra-Ocular Tension.

Softening of the eye is quite common as a secondary affection. The most common causes are detachment oi the retina and irido-cyclitis.

Essential Phthisis: This is a rare disease, in which the eye becomes soft without known cause.

Section Three

Diseases of The Lids, Lachrymal Apparatus, Orbit, and Muscles.

Chapter Fifteen - Diseases of The Eyelids

Anatomy of the Lids: Each eyelid is covered by a delicate integument, which is continuous with that of the face, and is lined by a mucous membrane reflected from the eyeball. Between these structures, from without inward, are the fibers of the orbicularis muscle (which is the sphincter of the lid), the tarsus, which is a dense plate of fibrous tissue, the one in the upper lid being about ½ inch in width, the one in the lower being about ¼ of an inch in width. The tarsus is about an inch in length, and gives shape and strength to the lids. Attached to the one in the upper lid, at its superior margin, by an aponeurosis, is the levator palpebral superioris. This muscle is the levator of the upper lid. The Meibomian glands are imbedded in the tarsi, which are closely adherent to the mucous membrane. The cellular tissue of the eyelids is very loose. Along the free margin of the eyelids are "the lashes

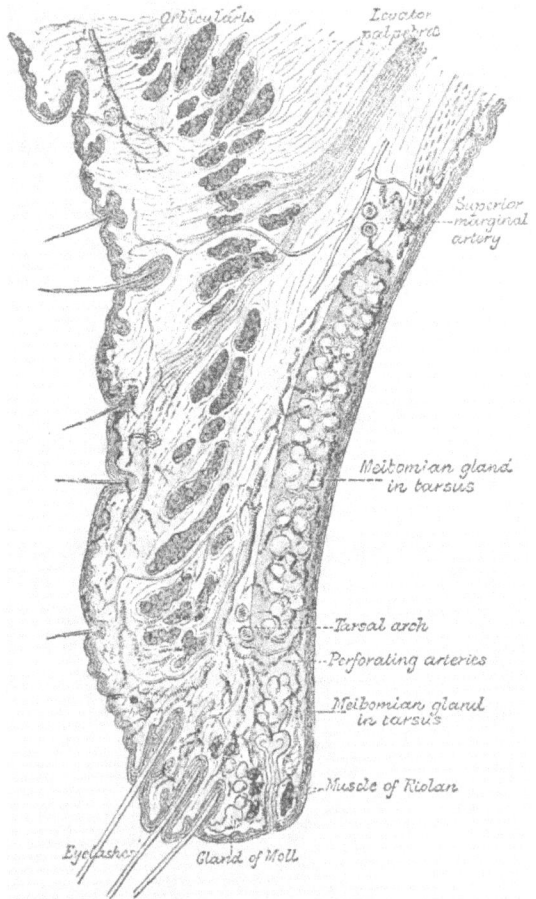

Section of Upper Eyelid.

or cilia. The blood supply of the lids is abundant. The nerve supply is from the fifth, the seventh, which is the motor nerve of the orbicularis muscle, and the third, which is the motor nerve of the levator palpebral superioris.

146

Blepharitis.

Blepharitis ciliaris, Blepharo-adenitis, Blepbaro-marginalis are the terms applied to inflammation of the eyelids. As a rule, the inflammatory changes are confined to the free margin of the lids. Its causes are parasites, irritating secretions from the conjunctiva, mechanical irritation, errors of refraction, etc. It is common in children who are poorly nourished and badly taken care of, being also common in the old and feeble. The symptoms are itching and burning of the lids.

Treatment: Correct any errors of refraction that may be present. Remove the secretion by softening it with a saturated solution of Bicarbonate of Soda. An ointment of Yellow Oxide of Mercury and Vaseline (5 grs.) will be found of value in destroying any parasite that may be present, and in keeping the lids clean and the secretion soft. No force should ever be used in removing the scales. The patient should be put on a nutritious diet, with plenty of fresh air and sunshine. The remedies that seem to be most frequently indicated are Pulsatilla 3x, Sulphur 3x, Arsenicum 3x, Hepar sulph. 3x, Antimonium tart. 3x, the general symptoms being the guide in selecting the remedy. Whatever remedy is given, it should be continued for a long time, as the disease shows a great tendency to recur.

Hordeolum, or stye, is a circumscribed suppurative inflammation, usually confined to a portion of a Meibomian gland and the tissue surrounding it. The symptoms are swelling of the lid, which is sometimes very marked; a red tender spot near the margin of the lids, and later, the appearance of a pustule. The trouble generally runs its course in three or four days, with a marked tendency to recur. Pulsatilla 3x is the remedy most frequently indicated, and should be given three times a day. Frequent bathing of the part in hot water will relieve the pain and swelling.

Chalazion appear as cystic tumors of the lid, filled with a gelatinous material. It is found at some little distance from the margin of the lids, and is an enlargement of an acinus of a Meibomian gland, with inflammatory thickening of the surrounding connective tissue. They are quite common in those who suffer from defective assimilation. Ant. tart. 3x is an excellent remedy to prevent recurrence. If the chalazion is of large size, with thin walls, it should be incised and the contents scraped out with a sharp spoon, so as to set up sufficient inflammation to cause obliteration of the sac.

Epithelioma is the commonest form of malignant tumor found on the eyelids.

Treatment: Removal.

Xanthelasma. This term is applied to yellowish-white patches of the skin of the eyelid. They are not dangerous, but most unsightly.

Treatment: Removal of the part of the skin affected.

Nsevi and angiomata are found on the lids.

Molluscum contagiosum is an affection of the lids, in which the sebaceous glands become hypertrophied. They appear as rounded tumors, with white centers, and contain cheesy matter.

Treatment: They should be incised and thoroughly scraped.

Syphilis may affect the eyelids in the form of chancres, gumma, and tertiary sores.

Treatment: That of syphilis.

Blepharospasm may be clonic or tonic. Its cause is irritation of the seventh nerve, which may be due to an affection of the cornea, iris, conjunctiva, or even the deeper structures, or it may be reflex from some other part of the body.

Treatment: Remove all source of irritation, and give Agar. musc. θ, three times a day.

Ptosis is a drooping of the upper eyelid. It may be a congenital anomaly, or it may be due to a disease affecting the third nerve, or to an injury. The congenital form can be corrected only by an operation. (See chapter on Operations.)

Rhus tox., Causticum, Arnica, Aeon., and Cimicifuga are the remedies to be consulted in the treatment of the other forms.

Ectropion is a turning out of the eyelids. It may be due to injury, paralysis of the seventh nerve, or to hypertrophy of the conjunctiva.

Treatment: See chapter on Operations.

Symblepharon is an adhesion between the eyelids and eyeball.

Ankyloblepharon is an adhesion of the edges of the eyelids to each other.

Lachrymal Apparatus.

The lachrymal apparatus consists of the lachrymal gland, which secretes the tears, and of a system of canals to carry away excess of lachrymal secretion. The lachrymal gland is situated in the upper, outer, and anterior part of the orbit. It is divided into two parts, with ducts, about twelve in number, which open in the outer part of the junction of the ocular conjunctiva with that of the upper lid. The arteries of the gland are from the lachrymal, and its nerve from the lachrymal branch of the ophthalmic and the sympathetic. The drainage system consists of the lachrymal canals; the opening of each is in a minute elevation, near the inner angle of the lids; these lead into the lachrymal sac. This lachrymal sac is located between the nose and inner can thus of the eye. It is continuous with the nasal duct, which is in the inferior meatus of the nose. Diseases of the gland are very rare, while those of the lachrymal passages are very common.

Dacryoadenitis, or inflammation of the lachrymal gland, in its acute form, is characterized by swelling of the outer part of the upper lid, with violent pain and chemosis of the conjunctiva with a muco-purulent discharge. A slight exophthalmus may be present, as a consequence of the swollen condition of the gland. In the chronic form, which is the more common, the only symptom that may be present is an enlargement of the gland. The acute form may result in suppuration, in which case an incision should be made on the conjunctival surface at the most dependent portion of the swelling.

Hepar sulph. 3x and Merc. sol. 3x are the remedies most frequently indicated.

Dacryops is a cystoid dilatation of one of the ducts of the lachrymal gland. The duct may be obliterated by the electro-cautery.

Fistula of the gland, which is generally the result of traumatism, may be cured by the electro-cautery, the fistula being thoroughly burned.

Tumors of the lachrymal gland, which, as a rule, are malignant, should be removed as early as possible.

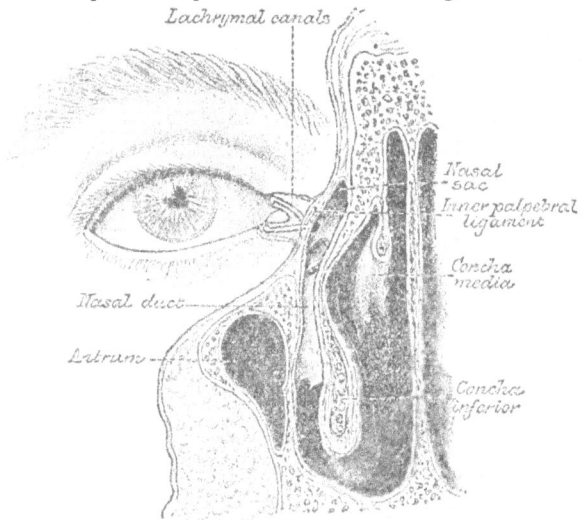

Section Showing Course and Relations of the Nasal Sac and Duct. (Merkel, modified by Quain.)

Diseases of the Lachrymal Passages.

These troubles are quite common, the great majority of them being due to catarrhal inflammation of the nasal membrane.

Dacryocystitis, or inflammation of the lachrymal sac, is characterized by violent pain under, over, and around the sac, and swelling of the tissues surrounding it. The eyelids may be swollen and the conjunctiva may be ©edematous. This disease is nearly always secondary to long-continued stricture of the nasal duct, leading to an accumulation of tears and mucus. Suppuration is very apt to occur in which case the lower canaliculus should be slit up and the pus evacuated. If the sac is allowed to break, a fistula is very apt to result, and this is very often difficult to cure. Frequent warm applications give relief. Hepar sulph. 3x is the remedy, a grain every hour. To prevent recurrence the stricture should be divided. (See Operations.)

Dacryocysto-blennorrhcea, or chronic catarrh of the lachrymal sac, is quite common. It is nearly always associated with stricture of the lachrymal passage. Its only symptom may be an overflow of tears. When pressure is made over the sac, if the canaliculae are open, mucus may generally be pressed out. Sometimes mucus finds its way through the nasal duct into the nose. Sometimes the patient has learned to press out the mucus, and in that case the history will establish the diagnosis. Stricture of the duct may exist without involvement of the sac, in which case epiphora, or overflow of tears, will be the only symptom. But remember that stricture is not the only cause of epiphora. Conjunctival, or corneal inflammation, or excessive secretion of the lachrymal gland, may be the cause. The careful introduction of one of Bowman's probes may locate the obstruction, but we do not advise this procedure unless all other means of relieving the condition have been tried. Dilatation of the lachrymal passage by probes, slitting up of the lower or upper canaliculus, and division of the mucous membrane of the nasal duct and electrolysis are recommended by most of the writers on these subjects. The results of all these procedures are very uncertain and unsatisfactory, as far as relieving the watering of the eye is concerned. Carefully selected remedies will be found to do more for both the cure of dacryocystoblennorrhoea and thickening of the mucous membrane than any other kind of treatment. Puis. 3x, Ant. tart. 3x, Hepar sulph. 3x and Merc. dulc. 4x seem to be more frequently indicated than any other remedies. Whatever remedy is given, should be continued for a long time.

Exostoses, or bony growths, may encroach upon the passages, giving

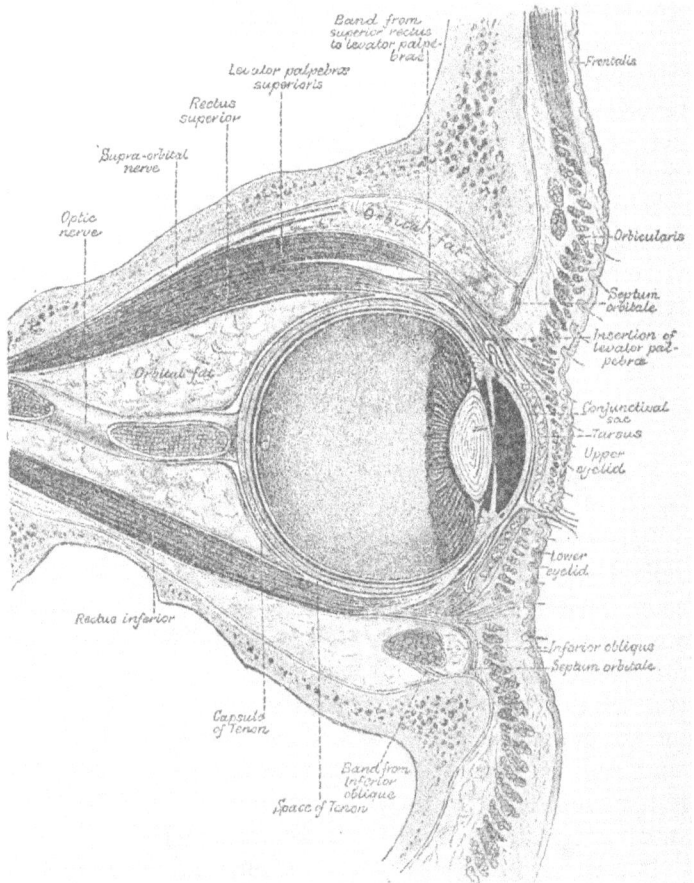

Vertical section of Orbit. (After Gerlach) magnified.

rise to an incurable stricture, unless the growth can be perforated or removed. Cataract operation should not be made on one suffering from dacryocystoblennorrhcea, as the corneal wound is almost certain to become affected. In all affections of the lachrymal passages the physician should bear in mind the importance of treating the nose.

Diseases of the Orbit.

The orbit is a bony cavity lined by periosteum. Surrounding the eyeball and its appendages is a collection of fatty, cellular tissue. The tissue forms a cushion for the eyeball, and surrounds all the structures contained in the orbit. Orbital cellulitis, or inflammation of the cellular tissue, occurs as a result of injuries, erysipelas, and in grave general diseases. Its symptoms are exophthalmus, or protrusion of the eye, and this is' generally directed forward; impairment of the movement of the eyeball, severe pain, swelling of the lids, and chemosis of the conjunctiva. When suppuration takes place, it is apt to point at some part of the conjunctiva. It is a grave disease, on account of the danger of extension to the eye, the venous sinuses of the brain, and the meninges.

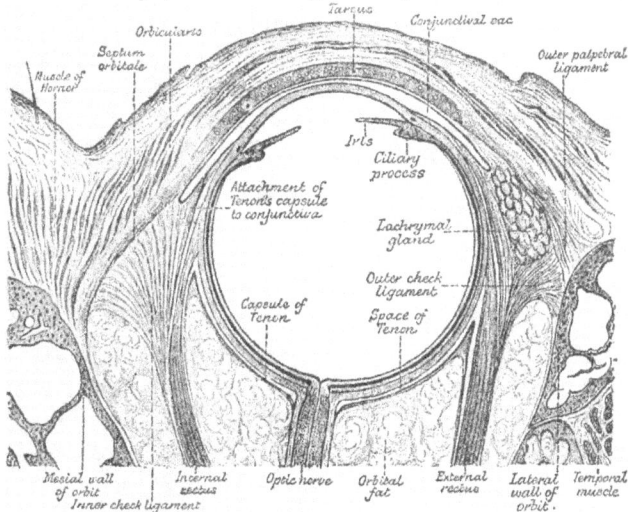

Horizontal section of orbit. (After Gerlach.) Magnified.

Treatment: Rest, warm applications, and, if pus forms, early evacuation by incision of the conjunctiva and cellular tissue. It is sometimes necessary to pass the bistoury deep into the orbit. Rhus tox. 1x is the most frequently indicated remedy, except when suppuration is imminent, then Hepar sulph. 3x will be found to be of great value. Periostitis of the orbit most commonly affects its margin. Caries and necrosis are apt to be a result of this trouble, from which children suffer more than adults. The symptoms of periostitis vary with the part of the orbit affected. If it be limited to or near the margin, a dull pain, with swelling of the eyelid nearest to the part affected, and a redness of the conjunctiva, with tenderness on pressure, may be the only symptoms. When the deeper parts of the orbit are affected the symptoms will be those of cellulitis, except that the protrusion of the eyeball is not apt to be directly forward, there being generally some displacement either upward or downward, or to one side or the other, if the inflammation be limited. The more deeply seated the disease, the greater the danger of the cellular tissue becoming involved. The general treatment resembles that of orbital cellulitis. Kali iod. seems to be more frequently indicated in this trouble, as most cases are due to syphilis.

Exophthalmic Goitre, or Basedow's Disease.

This is a disease in which the eyeball protrudes, and the upper lid is retracted and does not follow the movements of the eyeball on looking down. Associated with these symptoms, there is a rapid action of the heart and an enlargement of the thyroid. It seems to be due to a disturbance of the nervous system. For full description see works on neurology.

The attention of the oculist is called for when the eye protrudes so far that the lids cannot cover it, the result being that the cornea may slough. To avert this, the edg-es of the outer can thus should be denuded and sewn together, so that the palpebral aperture may be diminished and the cornea covered. The operation is called tarsorrhaphy.

Tumors of the orbit may be of three kinds — solid, cystic, or pulsating. The solid may be malignant or benign. They should be removed at the earliest possible date. A simple incision may be sufficient to obliterate a cystic tumor. The pulsating tumors are generally the result of a rupture of the internal carotid, in the cavernous sinus, giving rise to a communication between the veins and arteries. Pulsation of the eyeball may be felt, and a murmur may be heard with the stethoscope. This condition must be distinguished from other tumors, as an incision of the aneurism might jorove fatal. The only operation that should be undertaken is ligation of the carotid artery. They sometimes disappear without treatment, and sometimes continuous pressure made upon them by a finger or an instrument may cause their obliteration.

Injuries to the orbit include fracture of its walls, penetration by foreign bodies, and luxation of the eyeball. Fractures at the base of the skull are very apt to involve the orbital plate of the frontal bone, in which case the optic nerve may be injured and atrophy result. Foreign bodies should be removed, and the wound disinfected. A luxated eyeball should be replaced, and a pressure bandage applied to the eye. Arnica 3x and Aconite 3x will be found excellent remedies.

Affections of the Extrinsic Muscles of the Eye.

The muscles that move the eyeball are six in number — viz., the internal, external, superior and inferior recti, and the superior and inferior oblique. With the exception of the inferior oblique, they all originate at the apex of the orbit, around the optic foramen. The inferior oblique arises at the inner and lower marginal angle of the orbit. The tendon of the superior oblique passes through a pulley at the inner and upper marginal angle of the orbit. In considering the movements of the eye, this may be considered its origin. The internal rectus is inserted in the sclera, about 5.5 mm. from the margin of the cornea, at its inner side, in the horizontal plane of the eye.

The external rectus is inserted in the sclera, about 6. 9 mm. from the outer margin of the cornea, opposite the insertion of the internal rectus. The internal rectus rotates the eye inward, and the external rectus rotates it outward. The superior rectus is inserted in the sclera, above the margin of the cornea, about J.J mm. The inferior rectus is inserted in the sclera, below the margin of the cornea, about 6.5 mm. The action of the superior rectus is to turn the eye upward and inward, and to rotate it so that the upper part of the vertical axis is turned inward. By vertical axis is meant an imaginary line drawn from the superior to the inferior part of the eye. The action of the inferior rectus is to turn the eye downward and inward, and to rotate the eye so that the upper end of the vertical axis is turned outward. The compound action of these muscles is due to the fact that the origin of these muscles and their insertion are not opposite each other when the eye is directed forward. When the eye is turned outward sufficiently to coincide with the axis of the orbit, then the muscles act as elevators and depressors of the eye. The superior oblique is inserted in the superior and posterior quadrant of the eyeball. Its action is to rotate the vertical axis inward, and to turn the eye downward and outward. The inferior oblique is inserted in the inferior and posterior quadrant of the eyeball. Its action is to rotate the vertical axis outward, and to turn the eye upward and outward. The third nerve supplies all the muscles except the superior oblique and the external rectus. The fourth nerve supplies the superior oblique, and the sixth the external rectus. The associated movements of the eye are those in which the eyes are directed to an object in the median plane, or to objects in the lateral plane. When the visual axes converge in the median plane, the action that brought this about is termed convergence. Here the two internal recti act together to rotate the eyes inward, the other muscles acting so as to assist them in directing the eye to the proper point. When the visual axes are directed to a lateral plane, then the internal rectus of one eye acts with the external rectus of the other eye. In all probability there is not a simple movement of the eye in which all the muscles do not take part, either in antagonizing or assisting the principal muscle. These facts should be remembered in considering deviations in the movements of the eyes.

Strabismus, or squint: By this term is understood a deviation of the visual axes, so that they are not directed to one point. Apparent squint is present when the center of the cornea, through which the optic axis passes, forms an angle with the visual line of such an extent that the eye seems to turn outward or inward, depending upon which side the visual line cuts the optic axis. That this is not a squint may be proved by alternately covering the eyes when they are directed to an object, and then observing if any movement of the covered eye takes place. If there be no movement, then the squint is false and requires no treatment, it being a deviation of the center of the cornea and not of the visual lines.

Latent strabismus, or heterophoria, is a condition in which the visual lines are directed to the object, but only by an excessive amount of nervous energy. Its causes are many. Probably the most frequent causes are errors of re-fraction, especially astigmatism, general debility, reflex irritation, an undue difference in the strength of the various extrinsic muscles, or a difference in nervous innervation; malposition, or abnormal difference in the length of the muscles, are also factors, as is also difference in the visual acuity of the two eyes.

Heterophoria may be made manifest by using a test that either changes the character of the images received by the respective eyes, or by displacing the ocular images so that the eye will receive the image on its macula lutea, while the other eye receives the image on an excentric part of its retina. The mental impression of an image received on the macula will be projected into space, so as to occupy the position of the object, while the image received on the excentric part of the second eye will not, after projection, coincide with the object. For this reason the first eye is said to be the fixing eye, and its im-age the true image, while the second is said to be the deviating eye, and its image the false one. Esophoria is the term used when the eyes deviate in-ward. Exophoria denotes a deviation of the eye outward. Hyperphoria (right or left) is a term used when the deviation of one visual line is above the oth-er.

Two of these conditions may exist at the same time, in which case the terms Hyperesophoria and Hyperexophoria are used, the first being a devia-tion upward and inward, and the second a deviation upward and outward. Any of these conditions may, in some cases, give rise to severe nervous dis-turbances.

The practical examination to determine heterophoria may be made as fol-lows: The patient is placed twenty feet from a small flame — a burning can-dle will serve. Several glass rods, united at their ends and mounted in a rim that can be placed in a trial frame, are used to change the image of the flame into a long streak of light, which bears no resemblance to the flame. This test was suggested by Maddock, and is the most reliable of all the test instru-ments, of which there are a great number. This test object is placed in one side of the trial frame, the long axis of the rods being horizontal, a red glass being placed in the other side of the trial frame. The patient is placed in a line with the light, which should be at the same height as his eyes; he is directed to look at it, and if he sees the streak of light passing, there is no lateral devi-ation of the visual lines. If there is a space separating the streak from the flame, heterophoria exists. If the streak is on the same side as the test lens, esophoria exists. If it appears on the opposite side, then exophoria is the condition. The lens should be rotated so that the rods are vertical, and if the streak of light then crosses the flame there is no vertical deviation. If it be above or below, then hyperphoria exists, being either right or left, depending upon whether the streak is above or below the light. The measurement of the deviation is made by placing a prism over one of the eyes. The prism that corrects the diplopia measures the deviation, which is usually expressed in degrees. The same test should be gone through, with the test object at a short distance from the patient. Heterophoria found under these conditions is termed heterophoria in accommodation. These tests should be made several times at intervals of several days or weeks, as great variation may be found from time to time.

Treatment: First the prescription of glasses to correct any error of refraction that may exist, as the great majority of these cases will be cured by this means.

If the deviation is very great, or the proper glasses have been worn without relief, a prism may form part of the correcting lenses, its strength depending upon the amount of the error, which should not be fully corrected. All sources of reflex irritation should be removed, and the general health built up. If all other methods fail, and the examiner has convinced himself that the error is due to a shortened, or an over-long, or abnormally placed, muscle, then a very slight and carefully made tenotomy may be undertaken. The operation may be made several times until the error is corrected. As the operator's skill in correcting errors of refraction increases, the cases requiring tenotomy will be found to be fewer and fewer.

Strabismus, or squint, is classified into concomitant and paralytic. The subdivisions are strabismus convergens, divergens, sursumvergens, and deorsum vergens, or inward, outward, upward, and downward squint. Concomitant squint is distinguished from paralytic by the muscular power being unimpaired; this will be demonstrated by the eye moving freely in all directions, and by what is called the primary and secondary deviation. To make the test have the patient fix an object; then cover the squinting eye, quickly uncover the squinting eye and cover the fixing eye, and watch the movement made by the covered eye. If it be the same in extent as the uncovered eye, the primary and secondary deviation are equal, and the form of squint is concomitant. If the secondary deviation be greater, the squint is paralytic. In addition, the movement will be limited in the direction of the paralyzed muscle. Concomitant strabismus may be periodic, when the squint occurs at intervals of time; alternating, when one eye, then the other, deviates; or absolute, in which case one eye always squints. Hyperopia is the great cause of squint, which is nearly always of the converging variety. When due to this cause it occurs, as a rule, between the ages of two and eight years.

Diplopia is rare, and the sight of one eye, if the squint be absolute, is nearly always defective. It is supposed by many writers that the non-use of the squinting eye causes the sight to become defective, the term amblyopia ex anopsia being applied to it. Myopia and defective sight of one eye are the greatest causes of divergent strabismus. The upward and downward squints are very rare. The treatment of squint is to correct the refractive errors. This will often cure, especially if it be of the periodic or alternating variety. The correcting glasses should be worn at all times, except when the patient is asleep. If this does not suffice, tenotomy of the stronger muscle, or advancement of the weaker muscle, or both, will have to be made (see chapter on Operations).

Paralysis of the Ocular Muscles.

The muscles of the eyeball most frequently paralyzed are those supplied by the third and sixth nerves. The diagnosis of paralysis of the recti muscles, if complete, is easily determined by observing the limitation of the move-

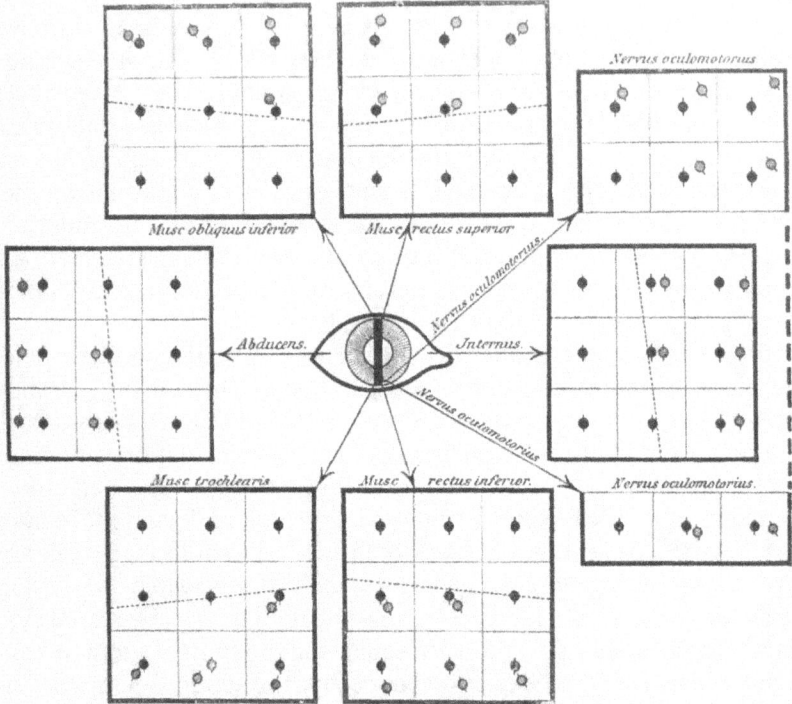

Relative positions of False and True Images in Paralysis of the various Eye Muscles.
(After Roth.)

ments of the eyeball, which is greater in the direction of action of the paralyzed muscle, and by observing the deviation of the cornea when an object is looked at; this deviation will be towards the sound muscle. Where the oblique muscles only are paralyzed, or where the recti are but slightly affected, the diagnosis is best made by determining the relative position of the projected retinal images of the fixing and the deviating eye. This may be done by placing a candle in front of the patient, and having him look at it; then a dark-red glass is placed over the properly directed eye, which is termed the fixing eye. To determine which eye fixes, have the patient point in the direction of the images seen with both eyes open. The eye that sees the object in its true place will be the fixing eye. The candle is then held about six feet from the patient, and directly in front of, and at the same height as, his eyes. Make a note as to the presence of one or two images. If two are found, note their distance apart, their difference in height, and whether one forms an angle with the other, and, if so, the amount of this angle. The candle should then be carried to the right and to the left several feet, and similar observations taken. It should then be carried to the upper and the lower fields of vision, which should be three feet above and below the middle field. The candle should be carried to the right and left in the upper and lower fields, as it was in the middle. The results are recorded on a chart, consisting of six spaces, in which the true image is indicated by an upright figure occupying the centre of each square, and the false image by a slightly different figure. The position of the false images, as they appear in paralysis of the different muscles, may be seen by referring to the chart, copied from Dr. A. Roth's.

Where only one image appears there is no double sight. It will be noticed that as the can-

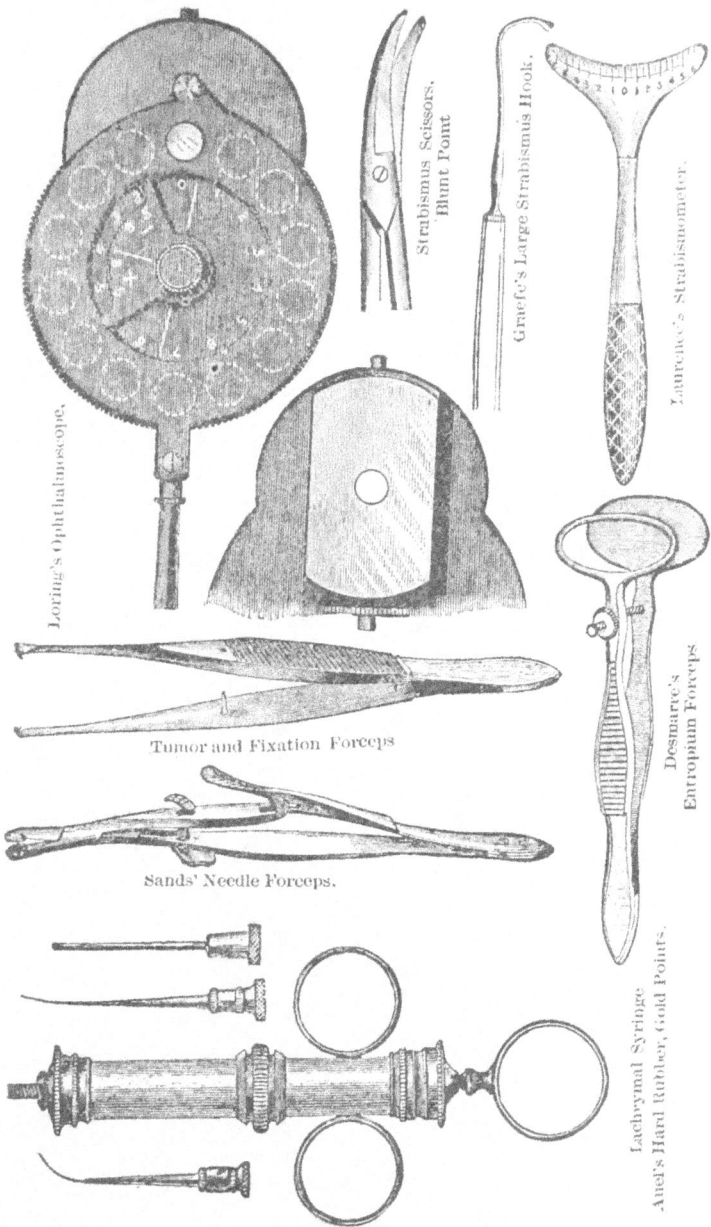

Loring's Ophthalmoscope.

Strabismus Scissors. Blunt Point.

Graefe's Large Strabismus Hook.

Laurence's Strabismometer.

Tumor and Fixation Forceps.

Desmarre's Entropium Forceps.

Sands' Needle Forceps.

Lachrymal Syringe. Anel's Hard Rubber, Gold Points.

dle was carried towards the paralyzed muscle, the distance separating the image increased. This is a general rule, and will indicate to which eye the defective muscle belongs. This brief outline only indicates the common forms of muscular deviation that are likely to be met with. To treat them all would require a very extensive work.

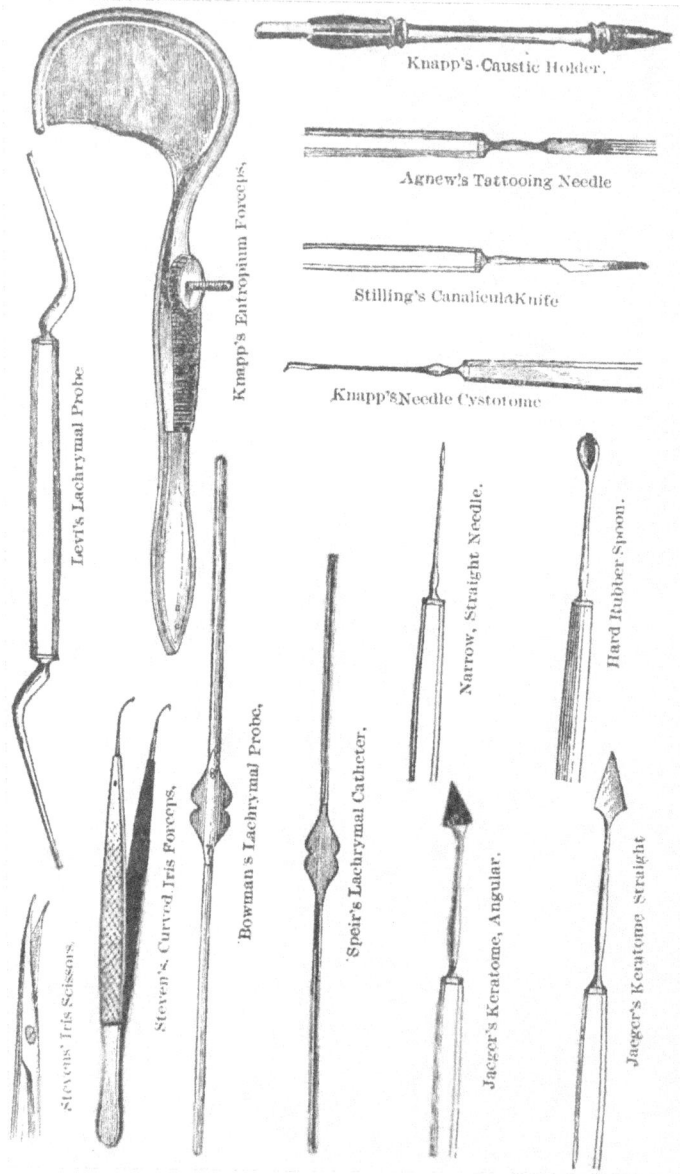

Knapp's Caustic Holder.

Agnew's Tattooing Needle

Stilling's Canalicula Knife

Knapp's Needle Cystotome

Knapp's Entropium Forceps,

Levi's Lachrymal Probe

Narrow, Straight Needle.

Hard Rubber Spoon.

Bowman's Lachrymal Probe,

Stevens Curved Iris Forceps,

Stevens' Iris Scissors,

Speir's Lachrymal Catheter,

Jaeger's Keratome, Angular.

Jaeger's Keratome Straight

My Cataract Technique. [1]

CHARLES C. BOYLE, M. D., O. ET A. CHIR.,
Surgeon X. V. Ophthalmic Hospital and College, New York.

MR. EDITOR: — You ask me to give you a few ideas upon the way I perform cataract operations. I do not know that I have any original ways in performing this operation.

I almost always perform the simple extraction, but if it is a case I think needs an iridectomy I make that at the time of extraction. I do not see the necessity of making a preliminary iridectomy, unless there has been perhaps a former iritis, and not always then if the eye is not irritable and there are not many adhesions.

In those cases where I have made iridectomy at the same time, there has been very little inflammatory reaction, perhaps even less than in the simple extraction.

In the simple extraction I have very little trouble afterwards, as a rule, but occasionally I run up against it as well as the others do. I do not believe I lose vitreous more frequently than do those who perform the iridectomy. Of course, in the simple you take the chances of a prolapsed iris, but it does not occur often, and then it is only partial. I always treat a prolapse by burning it two or three weeks after operation with the galvanocautery; this can be done as often as necessary, it has no inflammatory reaction to speak of.

The great mistake that I think a great many make after cataract operation is to want to look at the eye too soon; I generally wait until the fourth, fifth or sixth day. unless there are some symptoms indicating trouble. Some adhesion of the iris and capsule will then ensue. This is frequently the case, but it does no harm. These adhesions may be torn away with a mydriatic, or if that fails, the capsule can be divided, making a better pupil, sometimes, than the ordinary larger one. In case there has been an iridectomy I do not think it makes so much difference, but in simple extraction if you look at the eye too soon — that is before the wound has closed — you are apt to have a prolapse of the iris afterwards.

I do not think it advisable to use a mydriatic in simple extraction before the fourth day, even if the wound has closed — that is if the wound is in the cornea away from the periphery — because the iris will sometimes be drawn up against the inside of the wound and become adherent. But if the top of the wound is at the corneoscleral junction there is no danger of the iris adhering.

I used to finish my incision in the upper part of the cornea about one or two millimeters from the corneoscleral edge, but now I come out at the junction, or a little within the sclera, making a little flap of conjunctiva. The wound heals quicker and there is less astigmia afterwards. My puncture and counter puncture are about a millimeter from the corneal edge in the sclera.

I divide my capsule generally at the upper periphery; this lets the capsule act as a sac to retain what remains of the cortical substance, causing less irritation than if these remnants were floating around in the anterior chamber.

In operating I rarely use the speculum or foreceps, but I use my thumb to pull down or up the eyelid, and steady the eyeball by my forefinger while an assistant retracts the other lid. I am not ambidextrous; for the right eye I stand at the head of my patient, and for the left eye at his or her left side.

I flush the eye before and after the operation with a weak bichloride solution (1:ioooo) followed by boric acid, dress with gauze and cotton pads held in place by adhesive straps.

In this operation I do not always consider the loss of vitreous a serious matter, although of course I would rather not have it; the mere presence of a fluid vitreous shows you that you have not a normal condition to deal with. If you have a prolapse of a normal jellylike vitreous, I think the less you meddle with it the better; do not try to replace it or to cut it off, but close the eye and bandage as soon as possible — it will be cut off or absorbed in the process of healing with very little trouble.

If excessive loss of vitreous precedes extraction and the lens drops back, instead of hunting for it with the wire loop I press it out; pressure being made on lower part of the eyeball thru the eyelid by the thumb. Excessive loss of vitreous is replaced by injection of sterile normal salt solution.

49 W. 37th Street.

[1] Written expressly for this Journal.

Chapter Sixteen – Eye Operations

The description of operations in this chapter will be limited to those which, in the author's opinion, have proved to be the simplest and most practical. A description of the historical and rarer operations, though of great interest, is excluded, owing to lack of space. To make operations on the human eye so as to obtain the largest percentage of successful results, requires perfect cleanliness of the instruments and applications that are used at the time of the operation and during the healing process, and of the hands of the operator and his assistants; also, that the part operated upon and the structures surrounding it should be free from septic germs. To obtain these conditions of cleanliness, the patient's face should be well washed with warm water and soap, and then washed again with a one-thousandth solution of Merc. corr. The eye should be opened and flushed with a one five-thousandth solution of Merc, corr. Care should be taken to see that the edges of the eyelids and lashes are rendered free from scales and secretions, and that there is no disease of the lachrymal passages. The instruments should first be washed in boiling water, then in alcohol, then placed in a tray filled with a saturated solution of Boracic acid. If solutions such as Cocaine, Atropine, etc., are used, they should be freshly made with distilled water that has been boiled just before using. The hands of all that come in contact with the patient should be scrubbed with warm water and soap, and then washed with alcohol, and again with pure water, great care being taken to see that the finger nails are clean. The knives, scissors and needles should be very sharp, and free from rust or rough spots of any kind.

Operations may be divided into two classes: (1) Those made upon the eyeball, and (2) those made upon its appendages. The first class includes operations upon the conjunctiva and cornea, paracentesis, iridectomy, sclerotomy, and cataract operations. The second class includes operations on the lachrymal apparatus, canthoplasty, operations to correct strabismus, entropion, ectropion, ptosis, and symblepharon.

Operation for Pterygium: The head of the pterygium should be carefully dissected from the cornea, either with a small knife or fine pair of scissors. Incision should be made above and below the growth, starting from the corneal margin, and running diagonally to the base of the pterygium. This piece, which will be triangular in shape, should be removed. The conjunctiva above and below the wound should be loosened from the ball by snipping the subconjunctival tissue. The edges of the wound should be brought together with fine sutures.

Tattooing of the cornea may be done to conceal a dense leucoma, or to darken a thin one in order to improve vision, by cutting off the irregular rays that pass through the opacity. The operation is performed as follows: A solution of Cocaine is instilled, and, when the cornea has become insensible, the leucoma is pricked with a fine needle, or bunch of needles, directed diagonally to the surface of the cornea. Then a paste, made of India ink and distilled water, is gently rubbed into the wound, and the surplus washed off with pure water. No instrument that is likely to wound the conjunctiva should be used to hold the eye, because the ink will form a stain wherever the surface is broken.

Iridectomy, or removal of a part of the iris by excision. This is best accomplished under general anaesthesia. The operation is performed by making an incision through the cornea, then pulling out a portion of the iris and cutting it off. The place and extent of incision is determined by the purpose of the iridectomy. An iridectomy to relieve tension should be as large as possible, and at the upper part of the iris. The incision for this should be made with a large keratome, behind the sclero-corneal junction, just in front of the iris, the point of the knife being directed towards the center of the eyeball until it enters the center of the anterior chamber; then it should follow the plane of the iris, so as to avoid wounding the capsule of the lens. The knife should be withdrawn very slowly, to avoid a sudden escape of the aqueous humor. The iris forceps should be introduced into the wound closed. When they reach the pupillary border they should be opened, and a fold of the iris grasped and drawn out of the wound and cut off as close as possible; care must be taken that none of the iris remains in the angles of the incision. If a part of it be caught, it can generally be replaced by the rubber spoon that is used for cataract extraction; but if not, it should be drawn out and snipped off. Iridectomy for artificial pupil should be small, and made so that the opening in the iris will be opposite a clear part of the cornea — preferably at the inner and lower part. The incision should be small, and in the clear cornea about one millimeter from the sclero-corneal junction; upon the size of the incision depends the size of the piece of iris removed. The object in making the incision in the cornea is that, for optical reasons, it is not well to remove the iris close to its ciliary attachment. In other respects, this operation can be made in the same way as an iridectomy to relieve tension. After the operation the eye should be dressed with a light bandage, and the patient kept in bed for the first forty-eight hours. The bandage may be removed when all redness has disappeared. The eyes should not be used for work for at least one week from the date of the operation. Sclerotomy: This operation is made by passing a narrow cataract knife through the sclera, behind the cornea and in front of the iris, carrying it across the anterior chamber, and making a counter puncture in the sclera at the opposite side of the eye. The incisions are then enlarged by a sawing motion. A bridge of sclera must be left, connecting the two cuts. The knife is then slowly and carefully withdrawn. After-treatment the same as in iridectomy.

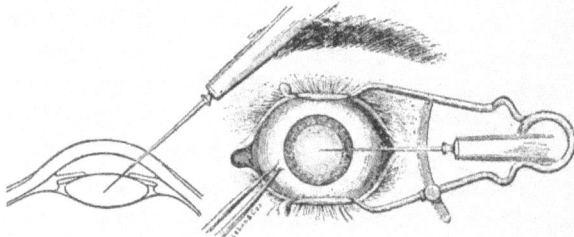

The Needle Operation

Cataract Operations.

In soft cataracts of young people the operation of discission, or needling, is performed to open the capsule and break up the substance of the lens. To perform it, the eye is held open by a speculum and the eyeball fixed with a pair of fixation forceps, and a discission needle passed into the anterior chamber through the cornea, and a small tear made in the capsule of the lens; this will allow the aqueous to enter the tissue of the lens, and cause it to become softened and absorbed. Care should be taken that the rent is not made large, for if a great amount of the lens matter escapes at one time into the anterior chamber it may cause an increase of tension, especially if the patient is not very young. This operation should not be made after the twentieth year. After that age, the case should be treated as one of hard cataract. Atropia should be used to dilate the pupil before the operation, and it should be kept dilated until the lens is entirely absorbed.

The operation for hard cataract, which gives on the whole best satisfaction, is known as the simple operation. The incision for this is made in the cornea, at about its upper third, with a narrow Graefe knife. The point of the knife is entered at the sclero-corneal junction, carried across the anterior chamber, and a counter puncture made at a point opposite the first incision; a to and fro motion will complete the incision, which should end slightly in front of the sclero-corneal junction. The cystotome should be introduced into the anterior chamber with its

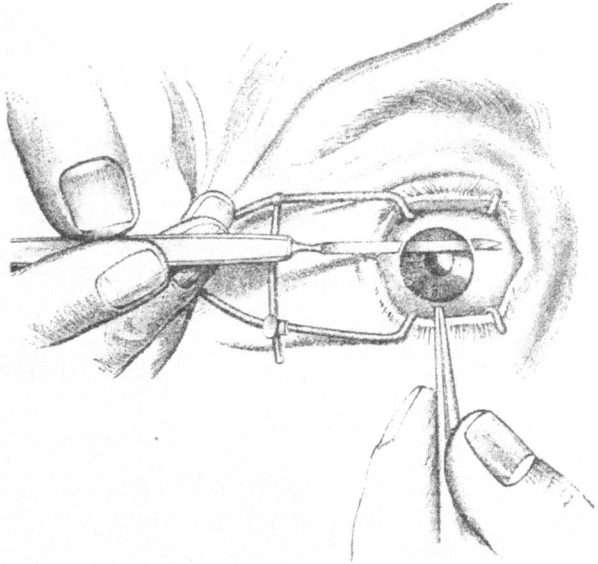

Cataract Operation.   Making Incision.

point directed to one side, through the pupil, and under the lower part of the iris; it should then be turned, with its point in contact with the capsule of the lens, and withdrawn, at the same time cutting the capsule well up to the corneal incision. Pressure is then made with the hard rubber spoon upon the lower part of the cornea, in a direction towards the center of the eyeball, so as to tilt the lens and make it engage the opening of the cornea. As the lens escapes, the spoon follows it upward upon the cornea and gently presses it from the eye. Any cortical substance that may remain in the eye should be gently coaxed on by stroking the cornea with the spoon, and removed as it appears at the cut. The eye should then be washed with a solution of Boracic acid, a bandage applied, and the patient put to bed. During the operation the eyelids may be kept open with an eye speculum, and the eye may be held still by a pair of fixation forceps, with which the operator should seize the conjunctiva at the lower part of the cornea by a deep firm hold. A solution of Cocaine may be used to render the eye insensible during the operation. The first instillation should be made fifteen minutes before the operation, and two more at intervals of five minutes, the eye being kept closed to prevent drying of the cornea. If the patient has very little self-control, general anaesthesia may be necessary; this adds a danger on account of the vomiting that may follow, during which the contents of the eyeball may be expelled.

Strabismus Operations.

Tenotomy of the stronger muscles may be all that is required to correct the deviation in strabismus. To perform this operation, the eye should be kept open with an eye speculum. The conjunctiva and sub-conjunctival tissue over the insertion of the tendon to be divided should be firmly grasped by the fixation forceps, held in the left hand. A vertical incision should be made through the conjunctiva and sub-conjunctival tissue, just in front of the forceps. If the effect of the tenotomy is to be very slight, the point of the scissors should penetrate but a small distance under

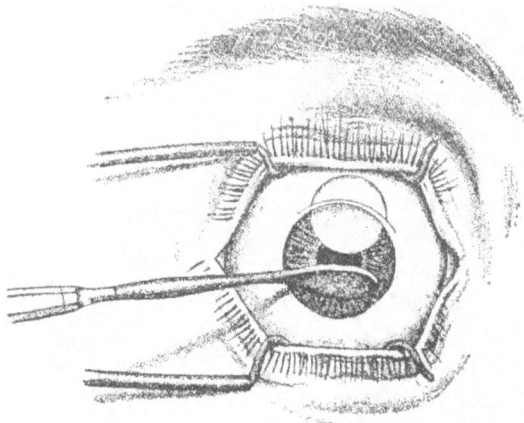

Cataract Operation.   Expelling the Lens.

the conjunctiva, and divide very little of the sub-conjunctival tissue. On the other hand, if the fault to be corrected is very great, the sub-conjunctival tissue should be freely divided. A strabismus hook should be introduced into the wound, and the tendon hooked up and divided close to the sclerotic. A smaller hook should then be passed around the place of insertion, and any remaining fibers of the muscle still attached should be taken up and divided. A suture should be used to bring the edges of the conjunctiva together. To some extent the effect of the operation can be modified by tying this stitch loosely or tightly. The simplest method for the advancement of a rectus muscle is known as Swanzy's operation. The muscle is exposed by making a vertical incision close

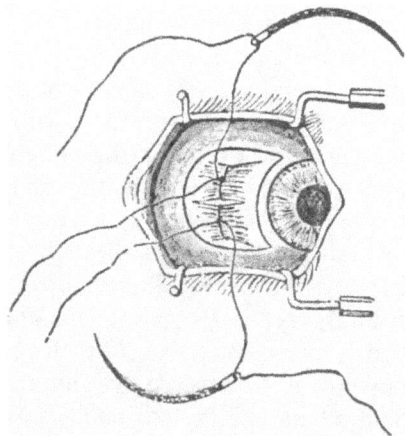

Advancement of External Rectus.

to the margin of the cornea and cutting off a strip of conjuctiva, about four mm. wide, parallel with the incision, passing a hook under the tendon and then passing threaded needles, one through its lower half and another through its upper half; the threads should be tied around the respective half of the tendon, long ends being left. The tendon should then be divided close to the sclera and the needles passed through the conjunctiva, above and below the incision, close to the cornea, and the threads tied. This will bring the several ends of the tendon close to the corneal margin, where a new attachment will be formed. The wound in the conjunctiva should then be stitched together. The stitches may, as a rule, be removed in five or six days. For this operation the local action of Cocaine will answer for adults, but for children general anaesthesia will be found necessary.

Slitting the canaliculus is a very simple operation, and may be made as follows: The edge of the eyelid is drawn outward, and the probe point of Weber's knife introduced into the punctual. The knife is then brought to a horizontal position and pushed forward until its point strikes the nasal wall. The handle is then elevated, with its edge upward, thus

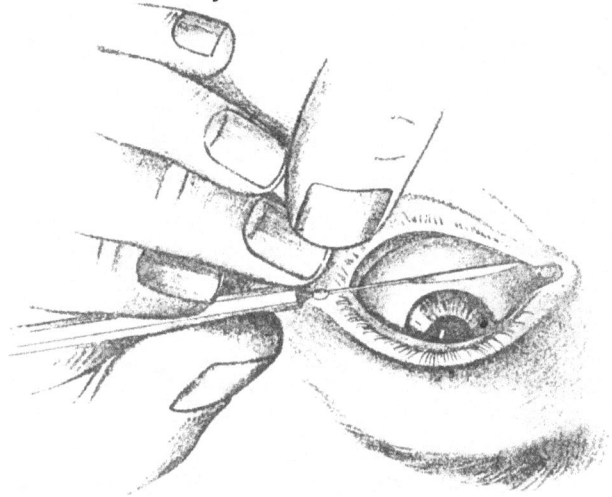

Slitting the Canaliculus.

slitting the canaliculus. Strictures of the nasal duct are best divided by Stilling's knife. This knife is pushed along the groove formed by the slit canaliculus until it strikes the nasal wall. It is then directed vertically, with its edge directed forward, and thus pushed down the nasal duct. The handle of the knife should rest against the brow, and the point of the knife should be directed a little backward and outward. No force should be used. Lachrymal probes may be introduced in the same manner as the knife.

Canthoplasty is made by cutting the outer canthus, and stitching the skin and mucous membrane together. Its object is to widen the palpebral aperture. The

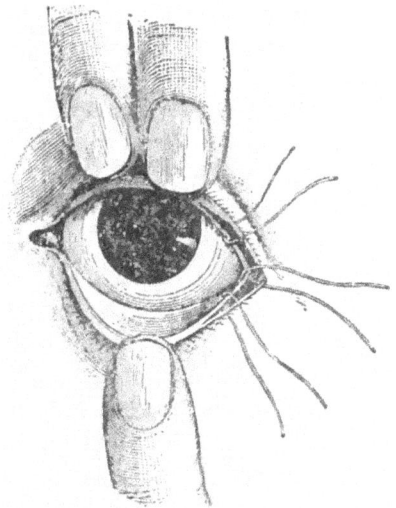

Canthoplasty

simplest operation for entropion is by removal of an elliptical fold of skin. The edges of the wound are then stitched together, so as to turn the edge of the lid outward.

Adams' operation is the simplest for correction of entropion in old persons. In this a V shaped piece of the lid is removed, and the edges brought together with two hairlip pins. When the entropion is due to cicatricial contraction, the scar tissue should be removed and the gap filled up by normal skin.

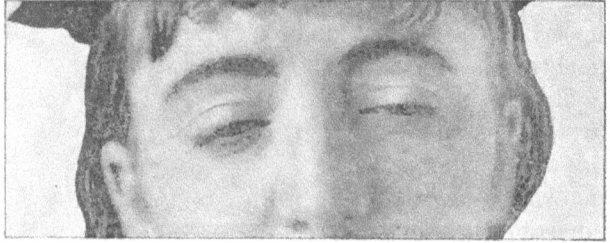

Ptosis.

Slight cases of ptosis may be remedied by removal of a fold of skin and connective tissue from the lid, and the stitching together of the wound. To correct symblepharon, remove the scar tissue and transplant a portion of normal conjunctiva, and stitch in the wound.

Enucleation of the Eyeball.

In this operation the patient should be anaesthetized, and the eyelids held open with an eye speculum, the eyeball steadied with fixation forceps, the conjunctiva over the superior rectus muscle incised, and the tendon lifted by a strabismus hook and divided. Then the internal, external, and inferior rectus are treated in the same way. If any part of the conjunctiva remains adherent to the eyeball, it should be divided, also any connective tissue fibers that may be found around the eyeball. The tendons of the oblique muscles may be then hooked up and divided. Then the eyeball should be made to pop out of its socket by pressure made upon the upper and lower lids. A strong pair of scissors, curved on the fiat, should be passed under the eye and opened as soon as they touch the optic nerve. They may then be passed further under the eyeball, so that the nerve comes well within the blades of the scissors, which should be pressed close to the eyeball, and the nerve divided. The eyeball may then be turned out, and any remaining fibres divided. The orbit should then be washed with a solution of Merc, cor., one to a thousand, and a pad of absorbent cotton placed over the lids and a firm bandage applied. In about two weeks' time the first glass eye should be inserted, which eye should be smaller than the one that is to be worn permanently; at first it should be only worn for an hour or two every day, until the socket becomes used to its presence. The patient should be cautioned not to wear the glass eye after it has become roughened in the slightest degree. It should be removed every night, and washed with alcohol.

www.ingramcontent.com/pod-product-compliance
Lightning Source LLC
Chambersburg PA
CBHW022039190326
41520CB00008B/652